Cancer Treatment and Research

Volume 163

Series editor

Steven T. Rosen, Duarte, CA, USA

More information about this series at http://www.springer.com/series/5808

Jeffrey Raizer · Andrew Parsa
Editors

Current Understanding and Treatment of Gliomas

Springer

Editors
Jeffrey Raizer
Department of Neurology
Northwestern University
Chicago, IL
USA

Andrew Parsa
Department of Neurosurgery
Northwestern University
Chicago, IL
USA

ISSN 0927-3042
Cancer Treatment and Research
ISBN 978-3-319-12047-8 ISBN 978-3-319-12048-5 (eBook)
DOI 10.1007/978-3-319-12048-5

Library of Congress Control Number: 2014956484

Springer Cham Heidelberg New York Dordrecht London

Printed on acid-free paper

Springer International Publishing AG Switzerland is part of Springer Science+Business Media (www.springer.com)

Contents

Epidemiology of Gliomas

Quinn T. Ostrom, Haley Gittleman, Lindsay Stetson, Selene M. Virk and Jill S. Barnholtz-Sloan

Abstract Gliomas are the most common type of primary intracranial tumors. Some glioma subtypes cause significant mortality and morbidity that are disproportionate to their relatively rare incidence. A very small proportion of glioma cases can be attributed to inherited genetic disorders. Many potential risk factors for glioma have been studied to date, but few provide explanation for the number of brain tumors identified. The most significant of these factors includes increased risk due to exposure to ionizing radiation, and decreased risk with history of allergy or atopic disease. The potential effect of exposure to cellular phones has been studied extensively, but the results remain inconclusive. Recent genomic analyses, using the genome-wide association study (GWAS) design, have identified several inherited risk variants that are associated with increased glioma risk. The following chapter provides an overview of the current state of research in the epidemiology of intracranial glioma.

Keywords Glioma · Epidemiology · Incidence · Risk factors · Ionizing radiation · Cellular phones · GWAS · Allergy

Contents

Q.T. Ostrom · H. Gittleman · L. Stetson · S.M. Virk · J.S. Barnholtz-Sloan (✉)
Case Comprehensive Cancer Center, Case Western Reserve University School of Medicine, 11100 Euclid Ave. Wearn 152, Cleveland, OH 44106-5065, USA
e-mail: jsb42@case.edu

J. Raizer and A. Parsa (eds.), *Current Understanding and Treatment of Gliomas*, Cancer Treatment and Research 163, DOI 10.1007/978-3-319-12048-5_1

1 Introduction

Gliomas represent 31 % of all brain and central nervous system (CNS) tumors diagnosed in the United States, and 81 % of malignant brain and CNS tumors [1]. These tumors are classified using World Health Organization (WHO) grade criteria, and can be classified into multiple specific histologic subtypes. The most commonly occurring types of gliomas include: astrocytoma (WHO grade I–IV), oligodendroglioma (WHO grade II–III), and oligoastrocytomas (WHO grade II–II). Although gliomas are typically malignant, not all types consistently behave in a malignant fashion. The heterogeneity of gliomas (in terms of histology, grade, clinical outcomes, and genomics) increases the complexity of risk factor research in this tumor type.

2 Incidence

Incidence rates of glioma, i.e., the rate of newly diagnosed glioma, vary significantly by histologic type, age at diagnosis, gender, race, ethnicity, and geographic location. In general, gliomas are more common with increasing age, male gender, white race, and non-Hispanic ethnicity [2]. The most common type of glioma is glioblastoma (GBM), which ranges in age-adjusted incidence rate from 0.59 to 3.69 per 100,000 persons depending on reporting country/organization. Anaplastic astrocytoma (WHO grade III) and GBM are highest in incidence among those 75–84-years old, but oligodendroglioma and oligoastrocytomas are most common in those 35–44-years old.

Gliomas make up the largest proportion of malignant brain tumors, therefore reported overall brain cancer incidence rates should largely reflect glioma incidence. Incidence of brain cancer varies significantly internationally, as do methods of case ascertainment and surveillance (Fig. 1). Brain cancer incidence is the highest in Europe (Age-standardized incidence rate [ASR]: 5.5 per 100,000 persons), North America (ASR: 5.3 per 100,000 persons), Australia/New Zealand (ASR: 5.3 per 100,000 persons), western Asia (ASR: 5.2 per 100,000 persons), and northern Africa (ASR: 5.0 per 100,000 persons) [3]. It is lowest in South-Central Asia (ASR: 1.8 per 100,000 persons), sub-Saharan Africa (ASR: 0.8 per 100,000 persons), and Oceania (Excluding Australia and New Zealand, ASR: 0.5 per 100,000 persons). It is difficult to determine whether these differences are due to variation in data collection technique and/or coverage of surveillance methods, or are “true” differences in incidence. Incidence rates vary over time per registry (Fig. 2) and by gender, where males have higher incidence rates as compared to females. However, it is difficult to determine how much of these differences in incidence by registry are caused by “true” differences in incidence, as opposed to effects of data collection technique. Most registries note an increase in malignant

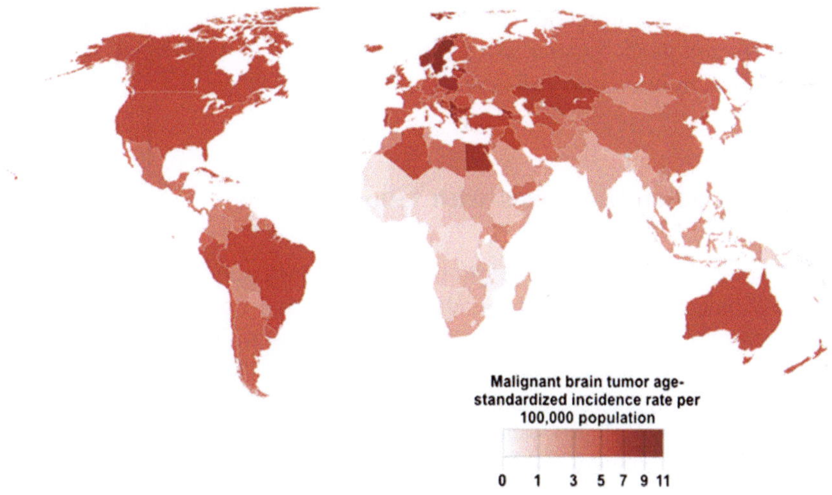

Fig. 1 Age-standardized incidence rates of malignant brain tumors (males and females combined) per 100,000 persons in 2012 by country (GLOBOCAN)

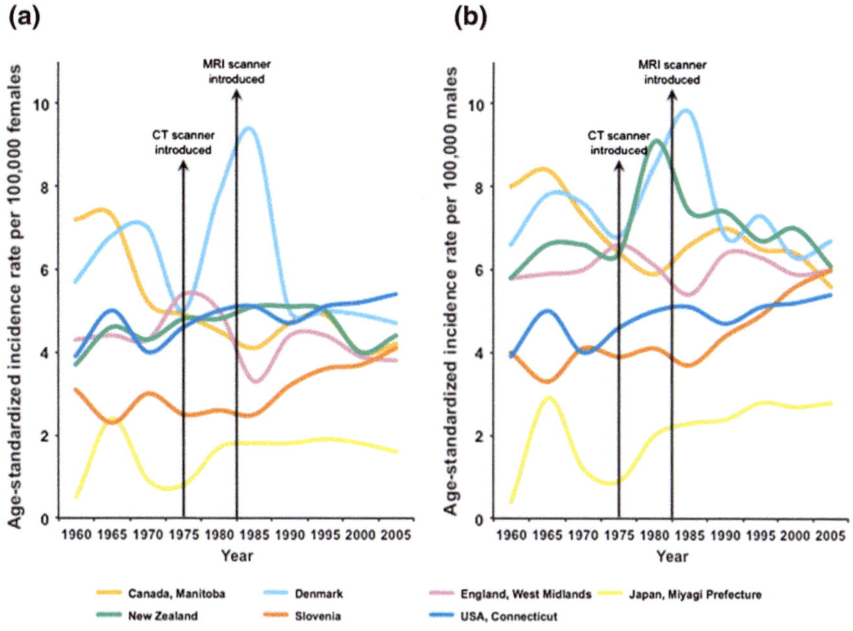

Fig. 2 Age-standardized incidence rates of malignant brain tumor per 100,000 females (**a**) and per 100,000 males (**b**) from 1960 to 2005 (GLOBOCAN)

brain tumor incidence from the mid-1970s to the mid-1980s (Fig. 2), when the use of CT scan and MRI became more common leading to a potential screening/ diagnostic bias in brain tumor diagnoses.

3 Survival After Diagnosis with Glioma

Survival time after diagnosis with glioma varies significantly by grade across all glioma subtypes (Fig. 3). GBM has the poorest overall survival, with <5 % of patients surviving 5 years after diagnosis [2]. Gliomas with an oligodendroglial component have increased survival when compared to those with an astrocytic component. See Fig. 3 for a comparison of relative survival from 1 to 10 years after diagnosis by selected glioma subtypes, from the National Cancer Institute (NCI) Surveillance, Epidemiology and End Results (SEER) system. Survival time is also strongly influenced by several omic markers within tumors, especially Isocitrate dehydrogenase 1/2 (*IDH1/2*) mutation, glioma-CpG island methylator phenotype (G-CIMP), O-6-methylguanine-DNA methyltransferase (*MGMT*) methylation, and 1p19q codeletion (See Chap. 4 for an in-depth overview of these markers).

The most conclusive and well-replicated prognostic factors for GBM are: extent of tumor resection, age at diagnosis, and Karnofsky performance status (KPS) [4, 5]. In 2004, the European Organization for Research and Treatment of Cancer

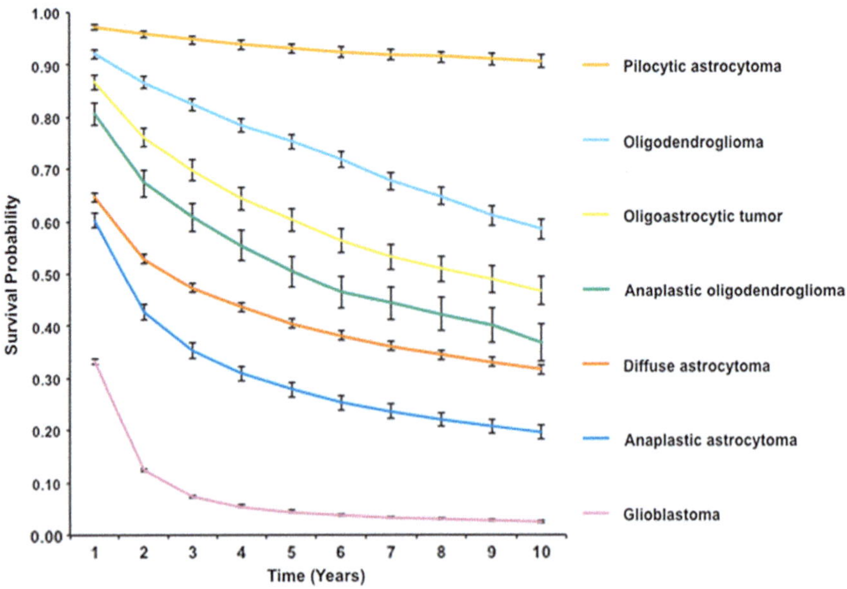

Fig. 3 One through ten year relative survival (with 95 % confidence intervals) for selected glioma histologies from 1995 to 2010 (SEER)

(EORTC)/National Cancer Institute of Canada (NCIC) 22981/26981 presented results from their trial that demonstrated a survival benefit for GBM patients that received concurrent temozolomide with postoperative radiation, with median survival of 14.6 months for those receiving concurrent therapy versus 12.1 months for those who received only radiotherapy [6]. This treatment has since become the standard of care for primary GBM (See Chap. 7 for more information on current treatment for GBM), and several analyses have found statistically significant increasing trends in GBM median survival after this was established [7–9].

4 Heritable Genetic Risk Factors

Several inherited, monogenic Mendelian cancer syndromes are associated with increased incidence of specific glioma subtypes, including: Neurofibromatosis 1 (astrocytoma and optic nerve glioma) and 2 (ependymoma), tuberous sclerosis (giant cell astrocytoma), Lynch syndrome (GBM and other gliomas), Li–Fraumeni syndrome (GBM and other gliomas), melanoma–neural system tumor syndrome (all glioma), and Ollier disease/Maffucci syndrome (all glioma) [10]. However, these monogenic disorders account for only a small proportion of glioma cases (<5 % overall). A small proportion (about 5–10 % of tumors) of gliomas occur in familial clusters, where a patient has a family history of glioma. First degree relatives of patients with glioma have a twofold increased risk of developing a brain tumor, especially when the patient developed the tumor at a younger age [10]. Linkage studies within these familial glioma clusters have not definitely identified high-penetrance risk variants [2]. A recent attempt to replicate the findings of these studies found that only genes that were also discovered using GWAS were replicable [11].

In the absence of a clear pattern of risk variants, segregation analyses have determined that genetic risk factors for glioma are best explained with a polygenic model [12]. Until recently, most of the studies assessing genetic variants associated with risk of glioma were candidate gene studies, focusing on genes thought to be involved in gliomagenesis. Since advances in technology that now allow for rapid whole genome genotyping, five genome-wide association studies of glioma patients have been conducted [13–17]. Together these studies identified seven genomic variants that increased glioma risk. The variants and their respective genes are: telomerase reverse transcriptase (*TERT*, rs2736100) [13–15, 17, 18], epidermal growth factor receptor (*EGFR*, rs2252586 [11, 15, 17, 19], and rs11979158 [11, 15, 17, 19]), coiled-coil domain containing 26 (*CCDC26*, rs55705857) [14, 17, 19–21], cyclin-dependent kinase inhibitor 2B (*CDKN2B*, rs1412829) [13, 14, 22], pleckstrin homology-like domain, family B, member 1 (*PHLDB1*, rs498872) [14, 17, 23], tumor protein p53 (*TP53*, rs78378222) [16, 24, 25], and regulator of telomere elongation helicase (*RTEL1*, rs6010620) [13, 14, 17, 18]. Four of these variants (*TERT, RTEL1, EGFR,* and *TP53*) increase risk of all types of glioma, while only three increase risk for specific grades and histologies (*CDKN2B*, *PHLDB1*, and

CCDC26). Both *CCDC26* and *PHLDB1* are associated with IDH-mutant tumors (predominately WHO grade II and III gliomas), whereas *CDKN2B* is associated with astrocytic tumors in general, WHO grades II–IV [2, 26]. The risk variant within *CCDC26* (rs55705857), though rare in the control population (<5 %), increased odds of developing glioma with a magnitude that is comparable to that conferred by early onset *BRCA1* mutations for breast cancer (OR: 3.1, 95 % CI: 2.5–3.9) [20]. The mechanism for increased risk associated with this variant is unknown [26].

Two of the variants that increase risk for all glioma types are in telomere-related genes (rs2736100 [*TERT*] and rs6010620 [*RTEL1*]). The single nucleotide polymorphism (SNP) identified within *TERT* (rs2736100) is also associated with increased risk for other types of cancer, including colon, lung, and testis. Telomere length has been associated with other types of cancer, but a recent case–control study has not found a significant overall association between this variant and risk of glioma [27]. The risk variants within these genes are more common among those with older age at diagnosis with glioma, which suggest that this telomere-based pathway may be a distinct mechanism of gliomagenesis.

Inherited mutations in *TP53* contribute to the development of Li–Fraumeni syndrome [10], and the mechanism for its contribution to gliomagenesis is well understood [2]. The risk allele identified via GWAS (rs78378222) in *TP53* is rare in the general control population (<1 %) and having this variant confers a 3x increase in risk for glioma. *EGFR*, *TP53*, *TERT*, and *CDKN2A/B* are genes that often acquire somatic changes during gliomagenesis, but more research is necessary to understand the relationship between germline and somatic changes in glioma [26].

5 Ionizing Radiation

Ionizing radiation can damage DNA by inducing both single- and double-strand breaks, and this DNA damage can induce genetic changes leading to cancer [28]. Exposure to therapeutic doses or high-dose radiation is the most firmly established environmental risk factor for glioma, and genetic factors influence the extent of risk from these exposures [2, 29–32]. Gliomas may present as early as 7–9 years after irradiation [32].

Studies of atomic bomb survivors were some of the first epidemiology studies to examine the relationship between radiation exposure and risk of malignancy. Preston et al. assessed the incidence of CNS tumors among survivors of the 1945 atomic bombings in Japan as a function of radiation dose. Tumors diagnosed between 1958 and 1995 among 80,160 survivors were ascertained using the Hiroshima and Nagasaki tumor registries, medical records, and death certificates [2, 33]. The risk for glioma was elevated, but not statistically significant, with an excess risk ratio (ERR) of 0.56 (95 % Confidence Interval [95 % CI]: −0.2–2.0) (Fig. 4).

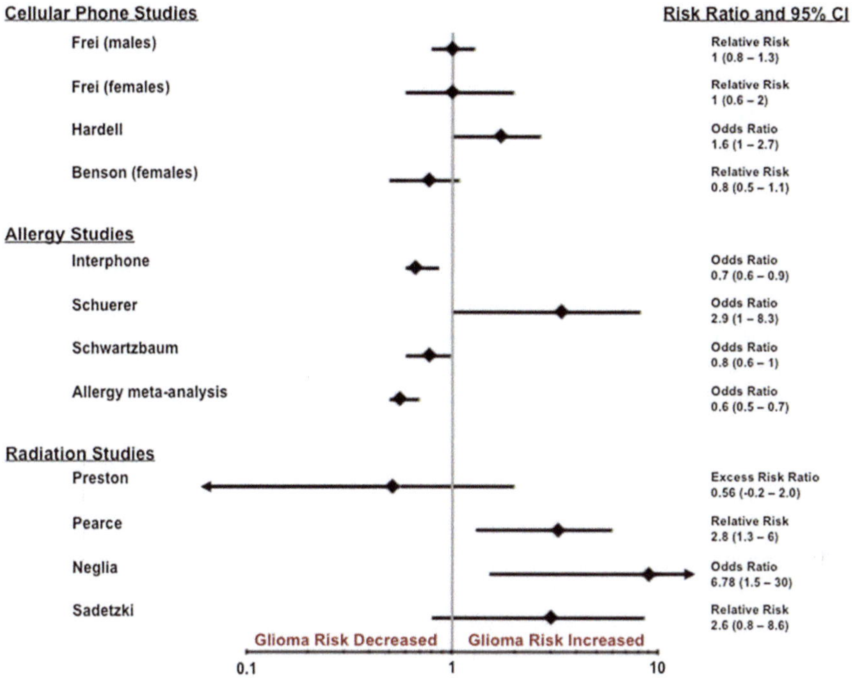

Fig. 4 Results of selected, recent studies of potential risk factors for glioma

A long running study of 10,834 individuals treated for tinea capitis with irradiation in Israel (mean estimated dose of 1.5 Gy) was reported by Sadetzki et al. With 40 years of follow-up, glioma incidence doubled compared to population and sibling controls (relative risk [RR]: 2.6, 95 % CI: 0.8–8.6) (Fig. 4) [34]. A dose–response relationship was observed, with ERR/Gy of 1.98 (95 % CI: 0.73–4.6).

Several studies provide evidence that therapeutic ionizing radiation is associated with an increased risk of glioma, especially in children. Two studies of the Child Cancer Survivor Study (CCSS) found increased risk of brain and CNS tumor in children treated with therapeutic radiation. In a retrospective cohort study of children ($n = 9{,}720$) treated for acute lymphoblastic leukemia (ALL) according to the therapeutic protocols of the Children's Cancer Study Group, between 1972 and 1988 [35] with a median follow-up of 4.7 years (range of 2 months to 16 years). Of 43 s neoplasms diagnosed, 24 were CNS neoplasms in children who had previously undergone irradiation [32]. This represented a 22-fold excess of CNS neoplasms, with 23 tumors occurring (including 17 gliomas whereas 1.06 were expected ($p < 0.05$). Neglia et al. also conducted an analysis of 5-year survivors within the CCSS cohort ($n = 14{,}361$) and identified subsequent primary CNS tumors in 116 persons (minimum 15 years of follow-up), including 40 gliomas (median latency of 9 years) [29]. Exposure to radiation therapy for primary cancer had an ERR of 0.33

(95 % CI: 0.07–1.71) and significantly increased odds of developing a subsequent glioma (Odds ratio [OR]: 6.78, 95 % CI: 1.5–30.0) (Fig. 4). In a case series of 1,612 children treated for newly diagnosed ALL between 1967 and 1988 at St. Jude's Research Hospital, Walter et al. [36] found 11 gliomas (10 WHO grade III–IV, and 1 WHO grade II) diagnosed as second malignancies. There was a significant association between 20-year cumulative incidence of brain tumor and cranial irradiation ($p = 0.015$).

Results of epidemiological studies assessing brain tumor risk associated with diagnostic imaging radiation exposure have been inconsistent. The range of effective dose for a single CT scan is estimated to be between 2 and 15 mSv. Though the effect of this level of radiation exposure is likely extremely small, many patients undergo repeat CT scans. In the last two decades, there have been dramatic increases in the per capita dose of diagnostic radiation, which now makes up approximately half the per capita radiation exposure. Recently, a group of radiation experts came to the consensus that the lowest risk of x- or gamma irradiation for which there is significant evidence of increased cancer risk is about 10–50 mSv [37]. Epidemiology studies of diagnostic radiation exposures have provided inconsistent results with respect to overall brain tumor risk. Two case–control studies of adults have demonstrated increased risks specific to gliomas [38, 39], most recently after three or more cumulative CT scan exposures to the head only in cases with a family history of cancer [39].

This potential cancer risk may be particularly relevant in children, whose brains are still in the process of developing at the time of irradiation exposure. Two recent cohort studies of children experiencing CT scans in Britain [40] and Australia [41] have suggested increases in cancer, including brain cancer, after childhood exposures to CT scans. In Britain, Pearce et al. studied the excess risk of leukemia and brain tumors after CT scans in a cohort of children and young adults. A significant positive association was noted between CT scans and gliomas (p: 0.0033), with an ERR/mGy of 0.019 (95 % CI: 0.003–0.070) [40]. Children who received a cumulative dose of 50–71 mGy had a significantly increased risk of brain cancer when compared to those that received less than 5 mGy (relative risk [RR]: 2.82, 95 % CI: 1.33–6.03) (Fig. 4). While almost 60 % of the CT scans were of the brain and the elevated risks observed for other solid tumor sites appeared to be dose dependent, these data were not consistent with an increasing risk per unit dose for brain tumors in children. The data related to risk associated with diagnostic radiation exposure is currently inconclusive.

6 Allergies and Atopic Disease

Allergies have been reported to be protective against multiple cancer types, including glioma [42]. Although the majority of reports have found an association between allergies and atopic disease (e.g., eczema, psoriasis, asthma, hay fever) with reduced glioma risk, some studies have reported the opposite effect [2, 43].

It has been suggested that the observed protective effect may be due to increased surveillance by the innate immune system for those with allergies, but this potential mechanism has not been definitively proven.

The initial approach for investigating the association between allergies and glioma risk involved analysis of self-report allergy history. Numerous case–control studies have examined the relationship between allergies and glioma risk. A 2013 study conducted by Turner et al. analyzed data collected as part of the INTERPHONE case–control study, which included brain tumor cases gathered across four continents, including Europe and North America [44]. The INTERPHONE study was composed of CNS tumor cases (glioma, meningioma, and acoustic neuroma) and controls recruited over a 4-year period starting in 2000. The analysis of the 793 glioma cases and 2,374 control subjects showed a decrease in glioma risk when any history of allergy was reported (odds ratio [OR] = 0.73, 95 % CI = 0.60–0.88) (Fig. 4). The protective effect persisted when data were stratified by allergy type (asthma, hay fever, and eczema), with hay fever being the most significant (OR = 0.67, 95 % CI = 0.53–0.86). A meta-analysis of 12 studies published between 1990 and 2009 that involved 61,090 participants (including 6,408 glioma cases) showed a reduction in glioma risk associated with allergic conditions (summary OR = 0.60, 95 % CI = 0.52–0.69, $p = 0.001$) (Fig. 4) [45]. The reduction in risk was maintained when data were stratified by allergy type of asthma, eczema, and hay fever.

A meta-analysis of 12 studies published between 1990 and 2009 that involved 61,090 participants (including 6,408 glioma cases) showed a reduction in glioma risk associated with allergic conditions (summary OR: 0.60, 95 % CI: 0.52–0.69, *p*: 0.001) (Fig. 4) [45]. The reduction in risk was maintained when data were stratified by allergy type of asthma, eczema, and hay fever.

In addition to stratification by allergy type, a more detailed view can be obtained by stratification based on glioma subtype. Scheurer et al. [46] and McCarthy et al. [47, 48] have both examined the effect of antihistamine or anti-inflammatory usage on glioma risk by grade and histologic subtype. Scheurer et al. found both protective effects and increased risk depending on glioma grade and antihistamine/anti-inflammatory drug usage. The lack of asthma or allergy history combined with less than 10 years of anti-inflammatory use was found to have the greatest protective effect for GBM (OR = 0.55, 95 % CI = 0.35–0.88). Antihistamine usage for 10 years or more was shown to increase risk of anaplastic glioma regardless of asthma/allergy history (OR = 2.34; 95 % CI = 1.20–8.34 with history and OR = 2.94; 95 % CI = 1.04–8.34 without history) (Fig. 4). McCarthy et al. found no significant differences based on grade for the effect of antihistamine use (low grade glioma [LGG] OR: 0.78, 95 % CI 0.46–1.33, vs. high grade glioma [HGG] OR: 0.75, 95 % CI: 0.57 –0.99), or reported allergy (LGG OR: 0.44, 95 % CI: 0.25–0.76 vs. HGG OR: 0.66, 95 % CI: 0.49–0.87) [40].

Use of self-report data alone is unable to conclusively establish a relationship between a potential risk factor and development of glioma. Another approach that has been used in attempt to elucidate the relationship between allergies and glioma is to examine serum concentration of the immunoglobin E (IgE), a common measure of allergic response; this measurement can be elevated in those with allergies [49]. In an analysis of pre-diagnostic serum IgE levels from 594 glioma cases (374 GBM cases) and 1,177 controls from Janus Serum Bank in Oslo, Norway, Schwartzbaum et al. found a statistically significant reduction in glioma risk (OR = 0.75; 95 % CI = 0.56–0.99) in patients with total IgE > 100 kU/L compared to those with total IgE ≤ 100 kU/L (Fig. 4) [2, 50]. Analysis of GBM alone showed reduced risk, but this difference was not statistically significant (OR: 0.74, 95 % CI: 0.52–1.05). These findings were in contrast to a prospective study by Calboli et al. that did not find a statistically significant association with elevated IgE (≥100 kU/L), but did find a protective effect of marginally elevated IgE of 25–100 kU/L [2, 51].

7 Cellular Phones

The risk of glioma associated with cellular phone use has been extensively investigated since the popularization of cellular phones in the 1990s. Several large-scale case–control studies have examined reported cell-phone usage patterns between persons with glioma and those without, and have found mixed results about the effect of cellular phone use on glioma risk [52]. The International Agency for Research on Cancer (IARC) conducted a thorough evaluation of the epidemiological findings of this research and classified radio frequency fields as a possible carcinogen (IARC group 2B) in 2011 [53]. This classification is largely due to findings published prior to this that demonstrate increased risk of glioma in heavy users (variably defined) of cellular phones. Also in 2011, the International Commission for Non-Ionizing Radiation Protection Standing Committee on Epidemiology reviewed the evidence presented by epidemiologic studies conducted up to that point, and found that the trend of these studies was against a relationship between cellular phone exposure and glioma risk [54].

Six studies examining the relationship between cellular phone use and glioma have been published since the IARC report: two cohort studies, one case–control study, and three studies comparing incidence rates over time [2]. Both cohort studies used cellular phone subscription records (in Denmark and the United Kingdom [UK]) and found no increase in glioma risk, including those who had used cellular phones for longer than 10 years or daily phone use. In the first of these cohort studies, Frei et al. examined 358,403 persons (including 3,664 glioma cases) in Denmark who had subscribed to cellular phone service prior to 1995, and found no statistical significant risk for both men and women with use over 10 years (Men RR = 1.0, 95 % CI = 0.8–1.3, Women RR = 1.0, 95 % CI = 0.6–2.0) (Fig. 4). Using the UK million woman study cohort, Benson et al. analyzed 791,710 women between 50 and 64, and found no statistical significant risk with greater than 10 years of use (RR = 0.8, 95 % CI = 0.5–1.1) (Fig. 4). A case–control study conducted by Hardell et al. using 593 malignant brain tumor cases and 1,368 controls found an increased risk for any use of cellular phone (OR = 1.6, 95 % CI = 1.0–2.7) and increased odds for heavy users (>2,736 hours of call time, OR = 2.8, 95 % CI 1.6–4.8) (Fig. 4).

Surveillance of trends in incidence of glioma over time is also an important way to investigate the potential effect of cellular phone use on these tumors. There has been a rapid increase in the use of cellular phones since their introduction in the 1980s. Currently, the vast majority of people in the world use cellular phones. Three of these analyses have been published since 2011, looking at trends in the Nordic countries (Denmark, Finland, Norway, and Sweden), the United States, and Israel [55–57]. All of these showed no significant increases in the incidence rates of glioma. These studies also compared current incidence rates to those that would have occurred with the magnitude of risk reported by previous case–control studies, and found that current incidence rates were much lower than predicted.

The scientific evidence used to produce the 2011 IARC report, as well as the scientific evidence reported since its publication does not support a significant association between use of cellular phones and risk of glioma. This exposure warrants continued monitoring and examination, as the potential risks of long-term heavy use, risk of use during childhood and adolescence, and length of glioma latency is not well understood.

8 Conclusions

Significant progress has been made in identifying potential risk factors for glioma, although more research is warranted. The strongest risk factors that have been identified thus far include allergies/atopic disease, ionizing radiation, and heritable genetic factors. Scientific evidence for an association between exposure to non-ionizing radiation in the form of cellular phones and glioma risk is inconclusive. Modern genome-wide "omic" technologies provide the opportunity to examine risk factors while accounting for the heterogeneity of gliomas. Further analysis of large, multicenter epidemiological studies, as well as well annotated "omic" datasets, can potentially lead to further understanding of the relationship between gene and environment in the process of gliomaneogenesis.

Conflict of Interest The authors report no conflicts of interest

References

1. Ostrom QT, Gittleman H, Farah P, Ondracek A, Chen Y, Wolinsky Y et al (2013) CBTRUS statistical report: primary brain and central nervous system tumors diagnosed in the united states in 2006–2010. Neuro-oncol 15(Suppl 2):ii1–ii56. doi:10.1093/neuonc/not151
2. Ostrom QT, Bauchet L, Davis F, Deltour I, Eastman C, Fisher JL et al. The epidemiology of glioma in adults: a "state of the science" review. Neuro-Oncol 16(7):896–913. doi:10.1093/neuonc/nou087

3. GLOBOCAN (2012) v1.0, Cancer incidence and mortality worldwide: IARC cancerbase no. 11 (Internet). (database on the Internet). International Agency for Research on Cancer 2013. Available from http://globocan.iarc.fr. Accessed 19 Feb 2014
4. Bauchet L, Mathieu-Daude H, Fabbro-Peray P, Rigau V, Fabbro M, Chinot O et al (2010) Oncological patterns of care and outcome for 952 patients with newly diagnosed glioblastoma in 2004. Neuro-Oncol 12(7):725–735. doi:10.1093/neuonc/noq030
5. Lacroix M, Abi-Said D, Fourney DR, Gokaslan ZL, Shi W, DeMonte F et al (2001) A multivariate analysis of 416 patients with glioblastoma multiforme: prognosis, extent of resection, and survival. J Neurosurg 95(2):190–198. doi:10.3171/jns.2001.95.2.0190
6. Stupp R, Mason WP, van den Bent MJ, Weller M, Fisher B, Taphoorn MJ et al (2005) Radiotherapy plus concomitant and adjuvant temozolomide for glioblastoma. N Engl J Med 352(10):987–996. doi:10.1056/NEJMoa043330
7. Koshy M, Villano JL, Dolecek TA, Howard A, Mahmood U, Chmura SJ et al (2012) Improved survival time trends for glioblastoma using the SEER 17 population-based registries. J Neuro-Oncol 107(1):207–212. doi:10.1007/s11060-011-0738-7
8. Darefsky AS, King JT Jr, Dubrow R (2012) Adult glioblastoma multiforme survival in the temozolomide era: a population-based analysis of surveillance, epidemiology, and end results registries. Cancer 118(8):2163–2172. doi:10.1002/cncr.26494
9. Johnson DR, Ma DJ, Buckner JC, Hammack JE (2012) Conditional probability of long-term survival in glioblastoma: a population-based analysis. Cancer 118(22):5608–5613. doi:10.1002/cncr.27590
10. Goodenberger ML, Jenkins RB (2012) Genetics of adult glioma. Cancer Genet Cytogenet 205(12):613–621. doi:10.1016/j.cancergen.2012.10.009
11. Walsh KM, Anderson E, Hansen HM, Decker PA, Kosel ML, Kollmeyer T et al (2013) Analysis of 60 reported glioma risk SNPs replicates published GWAS findings but fails to replicate associations from published candidate-gene studies. Genet Epidemiol 37(2):222–228. doi:10.1002/gepi.21707
12. de Andrade M, Barnholtz JS, Amos CI, Adatto P, Spencer C, Bondy ML (2001) Segregation analysis of cancer in families of glioma patients. Genet Epidemiol 20(2):258–270. doi:10.1002/1098-2272(200102)20:2<258:AID-GEPI8>3.0.CO;2-N
13. Wrensch M, Jenkins RB, Chang JS, Yeh RF, Xiao Y, Decker PA et al (2009) Variants in the CDKN2B and RTEL1 regions are associated with high-grade glioma susceptibility. Nat Genet 41(8):905–908. doi:10.1038/ng.408
14. Shete S, Hosking FJ, Robertson LB, Dobbins SE, Sanson M, Malmer B et al (2009) Genome-wide association study identifies five susceptibility loci for glioma. Nat Genet 41(8):899–904. doi:10.1038/ng.407
15. Sanson M, Hosking FJ, Shete S, Zelenika D, Dobbins SE, Ma Y et al (2011) Chromosome 7p11.2 (EGFR) variation influences glioma risk. Hum Mol Genet 20(14):2897–2904. doi:10.1093/hmg/ddr192
16. Stacey SN, Sulem P, Jonasdottir A, Masson G, Gudmundsson J, Gudbjartsson DF et al (2011) A germline variant in the TP53 polyadenylation signal confers cancer susceptibility. Nat Genet 43(11):1098–1103. doi:10.1038/ng.926
17. Rajaraman P, Melin BS, Wang Z, McKean-Cowdin R, Michaud DS, Wang SS et al (2012) Genome-wide association study of glioma and meta-analysis. Hum Genet 131(12):1877–1888. doi:10.1007/s00439-012-1212-0
18. Chen H, Chen Y, Zhao Y, Fan W, Zhou K, Liu Y et al (2011) Association of sequence variants on chromosomes 20, 11, and 5 (20q13.33, 11q23.3, and 5p15.33) with glioma susceptibility in a Chinese population. Am J Epidemiol 173(8):915–922. doi:10.1093/aje/kwq457
19. Jenkins RB, Wrensch MR, Johnson D, Fridley BL, Decker PA, Xiao Y et al (2011) Cancer genetics. Cancer Genet 204(1):13–18. doi:10.1016/j.cancergencyto.2010.10.002
20. Jenkins RB, Xiao Y, Sicotte H, Decker PA, Kollmeyer TM, Hansen HM et al (2012) A low-frequency variant at 8q24.21 is strongly associated with risk of oligodendroglial tumors and

astrocytomas with IDH1 or IDH2 mutation. Nat Genet 44(10):1122–1125. doi:10.1038/ng.2388

21. Enciso-Mora V, Hosking FJ, Kinnersley B, Wang Y, Shete S, Zelenika D et al (2013) Deciphering the 8q24.21 association for glioma. Hum Mol Genet 22(11):2293–2302. doi:10.1093/hmg/ddt063
22. Rajaraman P, Melin BS, Wang Z, McKean-Cowdin R, Michaud DS, Wang SS et al (2012) Genome-wide association study of glioma and meta-analysis. Hum Genet 131(12):1877–1888. doi:10.1007/s00439-012-1212-0
23. Rice T, Zheng S, Decker PA, Walsh KM, Bracci P, Xiao Y et al (2013) Inherited variant on chromosome 11q23 increases susceptibility to IDH-mutated but not IDH-normal gliomas regardless of grade or histology. Neuro-oncol 15(5):535–541. doi:10.1093/neuonc/nos324
24. Egan KM, Nabors LB, Olson JJ, Monteiro AN, Browning JE, Madden MH et al (2012) Rare TP53 genetic variant associated with glioma risk and outcome. J Med Genet 49(7):420–421. doi:10.1136/jmedgenet-2012-100941
25. Enciso-Mora V, Hosking FJ, Di Stefano AL, Zelenika D, Shete S, Broderick P et al (2013) Low penetrance susceptibility to glioma is caused by the TP53 variant rs78378222. Br J Cancer 108(10):2178–2185. doi:10.1038/bjc.2013.155
26. Melin B, Jenkins R (2013) Genetics in glioma: lessons learned from genome-wide association studies. Curr Opin Neurol 26(6):688–692. doi:10.1097/WCO.0000000000000033
27. Walcott F, Rajaraman P, Gadalla SM, Inskip PD, Purdue MP, Albanes D et al (2013) Telomere length and risk of glioma. Cancer Epidemiol 37(6):935–938. doi:10.1016/j.canep.2013.10.002
28. Wang LE, Bondy ML, Shen H, El-Zein R, Aldape K, Cao Y et al (2004) Polymorphisms of DNA repair genes and risk of glioma. Cancer Res 64(16):5560–5563. doi:10.1158/0008-5472.CAN-03-2181
29. Bondy ML, Scheurer ME, Malmer B, Barnholtz-Sloan JS, Davis FG, Il'yasova D et al (2008) Brain tumor epidemiology: consensus from the Brain Tumor Epidemiology Consortium. Cancer 113(7 Suppl):1953–1968. doi:10.1002/cncr.23741
30. Preston DL, Ron E, Yonehara S, Kobuke T, Fujii H, Kishikawa M et al (2002) Tumors of the nervous system and pituitary gland associated with atomic bomb radiation exposure. J Natl Cancer Inst 94(20):1555–1563. doi:10.1093/jnci/94.20.1555
31. Schwartzbaum JA, Fisher JL, Aldape KD, Wrensch M (2006) Epidemiology and molecular pathology of glioma. Nat Clin Pract Neuro 2(9):494–503. doi:10.1038/Ncpneuro0289
32. Ohgaki H (2009) Epidemiology of brain tumors. Methods Mol Biol 472:323–342. doi:10.1007/978-1-60327-492-0_14
33. Preston DL, Ron E, Tokuoka S, Funamoto S, Nishi N, Soda M et al (2007) Solid cancer incidence in atomic bomb survivors: 1958–1998. Radiat Res 168(1):1–64. doi:10.1667/RR0763.1
34. Sadetzki S, Chetrit A, Freedman L, Stovall M, Modan B, Novikov I (2005) Long-term follow-up for brain tumor development after childhood exposure to ionizing radiation for tinea capitis. Radiat Res 163(4):424–432
35. Neglia JP, Meadows AT, Robison LL, Kim TH, Newton WA, Ruymann FB et al (1991) Second neoplasms after acute lymphoblastic leukemia in childhood. The New England J Med 325(19):1330–1336. doi:10.1056/NEJM199111073251902
36. Walter AW, Hancock ML, Pui CH, Hudson MM, Ochs JS, Rivera GK et al (1998) Secondary brain tumors in children treated for acute lymphoblastic leukemia at St Jude Children's Research Hospital. J Clin Oncol : Official J American Soc Clin Oncol 16(12):3761–3767
37. Linet MS, Slovis TL, Miller DL, Kleinerman R, Lee C, Rajaraman P et al (2012) Cancer risks associated with external radiation from diagnostic imaging procedures. CA Cancer J Clin. doi:10.3322/caac.21132
38. Preston-Martin S, Mack W, Henderson BE (1989) Risk factors for gliomas and meningiomas in males in Los Angeles County. Cancer Res 49(21):6137–6143
39. Davis F, Il'yasova D, Rankin K, McCarthy B, Bigner DD (2011) Medical diagnostic radiation exposures and risk of gliomas. Radiat Res 175(6):790–796. doi:10.1667/RR2186.1

40. Pearce MS, Salotti JA, Little MP, McHugh K, Lee C, Kim KP et al (2012) Radiation exposure from CT scans in childhood and subsequent risk of leukaemia and brain tumours: a retrospective cohort study. Lancet 380(9840):499–505. doi:10.1016/S0140-6736(12)60815-0
41. Mathews JD, Forsythe AV, Brady Z, Butler MW, Goergen SK, Byrnes GB et al (2013) Cancer risk in 680,000 people exposed to computed tomography scans in childhood or adolescence: data linkage study of 11 million Australians. BMJ 346:f2360. doi:10.1136/bmj.f2360
42. Turner MC, Krewski D, Armstrong BK, Chetrit A, Giles GG, Hours M et al (2013) Allergy and brain tumors in the INTERPHONE study: pooled results from Australia, Canada, France, Israel, and New Zealand. Cancer Causes Control 24(5):949–960. doi:10.1007/s10552-013-0171-7
43. Rittmeyer D, Lorentz A (2012) Relationship between allergy and cancer: an overview. Int Arch Allergy Immunol 159(3):216–225. doi:10.1159/000338994
44. Turner MC, Krewski D, Armstrong BK, Chetrit A, Giles GG, Hours M et al (2013) Allergy and brain tumors in the INTERPHONE study: pooled results from Australia, Canada, France, Israel, and New Zealand. Cancer Causes Control 24(5):949–960. doi:10.1007/s10552-013-0171-7
45. Chen C, Xu T, Chen J, Zhou J, Yan Y, Lu Y et al (2011) Allergy and risk of glioma: a meta-analysis. Eur J Neurol 18(3):387–395. doi:10.1111/j.1468-1331.2010.03187.x
46. Scheurer ME, Amirian ES, Davlin SL, Rice T, Wrensch M, Bondy ML (2011) Effects of antihistamine and anti-inflammatory medication use on risk of specific glioma histologies. Int J Cancer 129(9):2290–2296. doi:10.1002/ijc.25883
47. McCarthy BJ, Rankin K, Il'yasova D, Erdal S, Vick N, Ali-Osman F et al (2011) Assessment of type of allergy and antihistamine use in the development of glioma. Cancer Epidemiol Biomarkers Prev 20(2):370–378. doi:10.1158/1055-9965.EPI-10-0948
48. McCarthy BJ, Rankin KM, Aldape K, Bondy ML, Brännström T, Broholm H et al (2011) Risk factors for oligodendroglial tumors: a pooled international study. Neuro-Oncol 13(2):242–250. doi:10.1093/neuonc/noq173
49. Gould HJ, Sutton BJ, Beavil AJ, Beavil RL, McCloskey N, Coker HA et al (2003) The biology of IGE and the basis of allergic disease. Annu Rev Immunol 21:579–628. doi:10.1146/annurev.immunol.21.120601.141103
50. Schwartzbaum J, Ding B, Johannesen TB, Osnes LTN, Karavodin L, Ahlbom A et al (2012) Association between prediagnostic IgE levels and risk of glioma. J Natl Cancer Inst 104 (16):1251–1259. doi:10.1093/jnci/djs315
51. Calboli FCF, Cox DG, Buring JE, Gaziano JM, Ma J, Stampfer M et al (2011) Prediagnostic plasma IgE levels and risk of adult glioma in four prospective cohort studies. J Natl Cancer Inst 103(21):1588–1595. doi:10.1093/jnci/djr361
52. Ostrom QT, Barnholtz-Sloan JS (2011) Current state of our knowledge on brain tumor epidemiology. Curr Neurol Neurosci Rep 11(3):329–335. doi:10.1007/s11910-011-0189-8
53. Baan R, Grosse Y, Lauby-Secretan B, El Ghissassi F, Bouvard V, Benbrahim-Tallaa L et al (2011) Carcinogenicity of radiofrequency electromagnetic fields. Lancet Oncol 12 (7):624–626. doi:10.1016/S1470-2045(11)70147-4
54. Swerdlow AJ, Feychting M, Green AC, Leeka Kheifets LK, Savitz DA (2011) International commission for non-ionizing radiation protection standing committee on e. mobile phones, brain tumors, and the interphone study: where are we now? Environ Health Perspect 119 (11):1534–1538. doi:10.1289/ehp.1103693
55. Deltour I, Auvinen A, Feychting M, Johansen C, Klaeboe L, Sankila R et al (2012) Mobile phone use and incidence of glioma in the Nordic Countries 1979–2008: consistency check. Epidemiology 23(2):301–307. doi:10.1097/EDE.0b013e3182448295
56. Little MP, Rajaraman P, Curtis RE, Devesa SS, Inskip PD, Check DP et al (2012) Mobile phone use and glioma risk: comparison of epidemiological study results with incidence trends in the United States. BMJ 344:e1147. doi:10.1136/bmj.e1147
57. Barchana M, Margaliot M, Liphshitz I (2012) Changes in brain glioma incidence and laterality correlates with use of mobile phones—a nationwide population based study in Israel. Asian Pac J Cancer Prev 13(11):5857–5863

Glioma Biology and Molecular Markers

Adam L. Cohen and Howard Colman

Abstract The tumors classified as gliomas include a wide variety of histologies including the more common (astrocytoma, glioblastoma), as well as the less common histologies (oligodendroglioma, mixed oligoastrocytoma, pilocytic astrocytoma). Recent efforts at comprehensive genetic characterization of various primary brain tumor types have identified a number of common alterations and pathways common to multiple tumor types. Common pathways in glioma biology include growth factor receptor tyrosine kinases and their downstream signaling via the MAP kinase cascade or PI3K signaling, loss of apoptosis through p53, cell cycle regulation, angiogenesis via VEGF signaling, and invasion. However, in addition to these common general pathway alterations, a number of specific alterations have been identified in particular tumor types, and a number of these have direct therapeutic implications. These include mutations or fusions in the BRAF gene seen in pilocytic astrocytomas (and gangliogliomas). In oligodendrogliomas, mutations in IDH1 and codeletion of chromosomes 1p and 19q are associated with improved survival with upfront use of combined chemotherapy and radiation, and these tumors also have unique mutations of CIC and FUBP1 genes. Low grade gliomas are increasingly seen to be divided into two groups based on IDH mutation status, with astrocytomas developing through IDH mutation followed by p53 mutation, while poor prognosis low grade gliomas and primary glioblastomas (GBMs) are characterized by EGFR amplification, loss of PTEN, and loss of cyclin-dependent kinase inhibitors. GBMs can be further characterized based on gene expression and gene methylation patterns into three or four distinct subgroups. Prognostic markers in diffuse gliomas include IDH mutation, 1p/19q codeletion, and MGMT methylation, and MGMT is also a predictive marker in elderly patients with glioblastoma treated with temozolomide monotherapy.

Keywords Astrocytoma · Glioblastoma · Oligodendroglioma · Pilocytic astrocytoma · IDH1 · EGFR · BRAF · 1p/19q codeletion · MGMT methylation

A.L. Cohen (✉) · H. Colman
Huntsman Cancer Institute, 2000 Circle of Hope, 84112 Salt Lake City, UT
e-mail: adam.cohen@hci.utah.edu

H. Colman
e-mail: howard.colman@hci.utah.edu

J. Raizer and A. Parsa (eds.), *Current Understanding and Treatment of Gliomas*,
Cancer Treatment and Research 163, DOI 10.1007/978-3-319-12048-5_2

Contents

1 Introduction

Gliomas are the most common primary brain tumor in adults, affecting about 20,000 people in the US each year [14]. Pathologically, gliomas are divided into astrocytomas, oligodendrogliomas, and mixed oligoastrocytomas based on histopathologic appearance. Most gliomas are astrocytic (82 %), followed by unspecified gliomas (7 %), oligodendroglial tumors (6 %), and mixed oligoastrocytomas (3 %) [14]. However, it is now understood that these histologies include a heterogeneous group of tumors with distinct molecular ontology and biology. Molecular classification has allowed for the identification of prognostic and predictive markers for some types of gliomas, and molecular subclasses are becoming increasingly important in the clinical classification and treatment of gliomas.

2 Histology

The 2007 World Health Organization classification recognizes three types and four grades of gliomas based on their microscopic appearance [45]. Grade 1, or pilocytic, astrocytomas are noninvasive tumors found primarily in children. Diffuse gliomas include astrocytomas, oligodendrogliomas. Grade 4 astrocytomas are called glioblastomas (GBMs). While some gliomas are mixed and have areas consistent with more than one type of histology, some investigators hypothesize that the different tumor types arise from different cells of origin and specific molecular alterations. Oligodendrogliomas probably arise from oligodendroglial precursor cells [44, 54, 72]. Radial glial cells have been proposed to be the cell of origin of ependymomas [74]. The cell of origin of astrocytomas has been proposed to be reactive astrocytes of the subventricular zone (for *NF1* and *PDGF*-driven astrocytomas), neural progenitor cells of the frontal lobe (for IDH-mutant astrocytomas), and neural stem cells/ progenitor cells in the subventricular zone [1, 22, 41].

3 Important Pathways in Glioma Biology

3.1 *RTK/RAS/PI(3K), P53, Rb*

Publications from the Cancer Genome Atlas (TCGA) effort showed that more than three quarters of GBMs have alterations, including deletions, amplifications, or mutations, in three pathways: growth factor downstream signaling, particularly through the phosphatidyl inosital-3-kinase (PI3K) pathway, apoptosis regulation via p53 signaling, and cell cycle regulation via cyclin-dependant kinases and retinoblastoma 1 signaling [75]. Alterations in growth factor receptor/PI3K/MAPK signaling can include amplification of the epidermal growth factor receptor (*EGFR/erbB1*), platelet derived growth factor receptor (*PDGFR*), or *MET* genes or mutation in *EGFR* or the *HER2/erbB2* receptor gene. Mutations in *EGFR*, particularly the EGFRvIII variant in which most of the extracellular domain is deleted, occur in 25–30 % of GBM [29, 76]. Downstream signaling from growth factor receptors can be activated by loss or mutation in the neurofibromatosis 1 gene (*NF1*), mutations in *KRAS*, mutations in *PIK3CA* (the gene for *PI3K*), and deletion or loss of heterozygosity of *PTEN,* the inhibitor of PI3K [75]. Although about one-third of GBM can have mutation or deletion of *TP53*, loss of p53 function can also be obtained through amplification of *MDM2* or *MDM4* [8]. Lastly, cell cycle regulation is disrupted through mutation or deletion of the cell cycle inhibitors *CDKN2A*, *CDKN2B*, and *CDKN2C* as well as less frequent amplifications in cyclins and cyclin-dependent kinases or actual loss of the *RB1* gene.Translocations and fusion proteins may play an important role in activation of growth factor signaling. About 4 % of GBMs have fusions of *EGFR* with *SEPT14*, which activates STAT3 signaling, and another 2 % have fusions of *EGFR* with *PSPH,* which regulates neural stem cell proliferation [17, 49]. In addition, approximately 3 % of GBM have translocations causing a fusion between the fibroblast growth factor receptor genes, *FGFR1* or *FGFR3,* and the transforming acidic coiled-coil containing protein genes, *TACC1* or*TACC3* [67]. There is in vitro and in vivo evidence that tumors with these fusions can be inhibited with appropriate tyrosine kinase inhibitors, but whether they are prognostic or predictive in people is not yet known.

3.2 *IDH Mutation*

In 2008, a multigroup collaboration using whole exome sequencing identified a common point mutation in the metabolic gene *IDH1* in 12 % of glioblastoma samples [53]. Further studies found that this mutation is present in ~80 % of grade 2–3 gliomas and secondary GBM [2, 7, 26, 37, 62, 84, 88]. Mutations in *IDH2* have also been identified in gliomas, although they are much less common and are mutually exclusive with mutations in *IDH1* [26, 69, 88]. All mutations identified to date have been a single amino acid missense mutation in *IDH1* at arginine 132 (R132) or the analogous residue in *IDH2* (R172).

Although initial reports suggested that the mutant IDH functions in a dominate-negative fashion by heterodimerizing to wild-type *IDH1* and impairing its activity [89, 92, 93], more recent in vitro studies have shown that the mutated *IDH1* protein acquires the ability to convert α-ketoglutarate (α-KG) to R(-)-2-hydroxyglutarate (2-HG) [13, 32]. These findings led to the hypothesis that mutant *IDH* is an oncogene and 2-HG is an "oncometabolite" [18].

New evidence suggests that by antagonizing α-KG, 2-HG competitively inhibits the activity of many α-KG-dependent dioxygenases, including but not limited to histone demethylases (e.g., collagen prolyl-4-hydroxylase, prolyl hydroxylases, and the ten-eleven translocation (TET) family of DNA hydroxylases) [16, 63, 87]. Profiling of GBM from the TCGA demonstrated an association between IDH mutation and increased promoter methylation (G-CIMP) [50], which generally results in transcriptional silencing of the associated genes [35]. Two recent independent studies demonstrated that the G-CIMP phenotype was not correlated with IDH mutation but that IDH mutation alone is actually the cause of the G-CIMP hypermethylation phenotype in diffuse gliomas [11, 40].

3.3 Hypoxia, Pseudohypoxia, and Angiogenesis

Gliomas often exist in hypoxic or pseudohypoxic conditions. The extreme example of hypoxia is pseudopallisading necrosis in GBM, when the tumor outgrows its own blood supply. Hypoxia causes the upregulation of hypoxia inducible factor (*HIF1a*), and *HIF1a* can induce new vessel formation and stem cell survival processes. *HIF1a* is overexpressed in gliomas, particularly high grade gliomas [43]. *HIF1a* degradation via the ubiquitin-proteosome system is also inhibited by alterations in prolyl hydroxylases driven by 2-hydroxyglutarate produced by mutant IDH. Thus, IDH mutation can result in a situation in which HIF1a protein levels are high (consistent with hypoxia) while oxygen tension is normal. This situation has been called "pseudohypoxia" and may be a major driver of biology in these tumors along with other consequences of altered proline hydroxylation.

Blood vessel formation in gliomas often takes the form of angiogenesis, driven by vascular endothelial growth factor (*VEGF*). *VEGF* is overexpressed in brain tumors, with increasing expression corresponding to increased grade [10, 56, 57]. Angiogenesis can also be supported by *CXCR4* signaling [90]. Alternatively, gliomas can coopt normal vessels, a process often mediated by angiopoietin signaling, or new vessels can be formed from bone marrow derived endothelial cells, in a process termed vasculogenesis [46, 60]. Glioma cells may even be able to transform into malignant endothelial cells [66]. It has been proposed that blockade of angiogenesis, particularly inhibition of *VEGF* signaling, may lead to increased glioma invasiveness, although this hypothesis remains controversial [38].

Invasion into normal brain is one of the hallmarks of diffuse gliomas and is one of the features making them incurable by surgery alone. Gliomas migrate along the secondary structures of Scherer, such as white matter tracks, neuronal tracks, vasculature, or subpial spaces [64]. Glioma migrations is facilitated by secretion of a variety of proteases, including matrix metalloproteases (MMPs), membrane type matrix metalloproteases (MT-MMPs), and adamalysins (ADAMS) [48]. Expression and secretion of these proteases can be regulated by TGF-beta and NF-κB.

4 Oligodendrogliomas

Oligodendrogliomas can be grade 2 (low grade) or grade 3 (anaplastic) [45]. There are no grade 4 oligodendrogliomas. One of the earliest steps in the development of oligodendrogliomas is mutation in isocitrate dehydrogenase 1 (*IDH1*) or 2 (*IDH2*) [84]. Mutation in *IDH1* or *IDH2* is followed by an unbalanced translocation resulting in loss of the p-arm of chromosome 1 and the q-arm of chromosome 19 [39, 59]. This translocation inactivates one copy of the Capicua transcriptional repressor (CIC) gene and the FUSE binding protein 1(*FUBP1*) gene [5]. Oligodendrogliomas then can develop a mutation in the other copy of these genes. Such mutations occur in 52 % of grade 2 oligodendrogliomas and 84 % of anaplastic (grade 3) oligodendrogliomas [31]. Whether these alterations are sufficient for oligodendroglioma development has not been established. The events involved in the transformation of grade 2–3 oligodendrogliomas have also not been established.

Codeletion of 1p and 19q is also a prognostic marker among all gliomas and among oligodendrogliomas, regardless of grade [91]. Indeed, mixed oligoastrocytomas with 1p/19q deletion have prognosis similar to oligodendrogliomas, while those without 1p/19q deletion have worse prognosis, similar to astrocytomas [30]. Moreover, 1p/19q codeletion is also a predictive marker among anaplastic oligodendrogliomas. Two randomized trials showed improved survival with the addition of chemotherapy to radiation for people with newly diagnosed anaplastic oligodendrogliomas whose tumors had 1p/19q codeletion but not for people whose tumors did not have this codeletion [9, 77]. Therefore, codeletion of 1p/19q, which can be detected by fluorescent in situ hybridization, is a clinically useful biomarker for oligodendrogliomas.

5 Astrocytoma Histopathologic and Molecular Classification

Grade 1, or pilocytic, astrocytomas are non-infiltrating neoplasms that occur mostly in children and adolescents but can occur in adults as well [45]. Pilocytic astrocytomas lack many of the mutations found in the diffuse gliomas. However, nearly all pilocytic astrocytomas have alterations in the *BRAF* oncogene leading to its activation, primarily by fusion with the *KIAA1549* gene [33]. Other mechanisms of RAF pathway activation include fusion of *SRGAP3* and *RAF1*, *BRAFV600E* mutation, in-frame insertion in the *BRAF* gene, or fusion of *BRA*F with *FAM131B* [12, 33, 34]. Activation of *BRAF* in neural progenitor cells is sufficient to cause pilocytic astrocytomas in mice and to transform human neural stem cells [21, 58]. How to target these alterations remains an area of study.

Diffuse gliomas can be categorized according to grade: low grade (grade II), anaplastic (grade III), and glioblastoma (GBM, grade IV). Traditionally, GBMs have been classified as primary or secondary on the basis of clinical presentation [65]. Secondary GBMs display evidence of progression from a lower grade tumor, whereas primary GBMs present as grade 4 at diagnosis. Secondary GBMs are predominantly found in younger patients (median age of ~45 years compared with median age of ~60 years for primary GBM) and tend to occur less frequently than primary GBMs, making up ~5 % of total GBMs [51]. Secondary GBMs are more likely to have mutation in IDH1 or IDH2. Despite the differences in their ontology, these high grade tumors are histopathologically indistinguishable [51].

In the 1990s, this clinical classification began to be correlated to molecular biology with the observation that amplification of the epidermal growth factor receptor (EGFR) gene and mutation or loss of heterozygosity of the TP53 gene was mutually exclusive, with the former being seen in primary glioblastoma and the latter being seen in secondary glioblastoma and lower grade gliomas [80, 83]. More recently, large-scale efforts have been made to identify the major genetic and epigenetic alterations and to define important molecular subtypes in GBM and lower grade gliomas [55, 79].

Gene expression patterns have been used by multiple groups to classify adult high grade gliomas into 3–4 groups [55, 71, 79]. The Cancer Genome Atlas (TCGA) identified four subgroups of GBM based on gene expression patterns, which were called Proneural, Neural, Mesenchymal, and Classical [79]. Individual gene expression subtypes were associated with specific genetic and epigenetic alterations. For example, proneural GBMs are enriched for the G-CIMP phenotype, *IDH* mutations, *PDGFRA* amplifications, and *CDK4* amplifications. Classical GBMs are enriched for *EGFR* mutations, particularly the EGFRvIII variant. Mesenchymal GBMs are more likely to have *MET* amplification and *NF1* mutation or loss and display increased angiogenesis, hypoxia, inflammatory infiltrates and inflammatory signaling pathways, including *NF-κB, STAT3, TGF-β* [3, 6, 55, 79] Secondary GBMs are virtually always Proneural, while primary GBM can be any of the subtypes. Most primary GBMs have *EGFR* amplification and deletion of the *PTEN* gene [8].

6 Prognostic and Predictive Markers in Astrocytomas

The two strongest prognostic factors in astrocytomas are *IDH* mutation status and grade [25, 88]. Indeed, prognosis for *IDH*-mutant GBMs is better in some series than that for *IDH*-wild-type grade 3 astrocytomas. The prognostic importance of *IDH* mutation is independent of other known prognostic factors, including age, and

MGMT methylation status [62]. However, it remains to be determined whether *IDH* mutation is a prognostic factor only or whether it is predictive of outcome to specific treatments or mechanistically related to treatment response. Small retrospective series have suggested that the response rate to alkylating chemotherapy is also higher in *IDH*-mutated grade 2 tumors than in wild-type tumors and that progression-free survival after radiation or alkylating chemotherapy is higher for people with *IDH*-mutated tumors than for people with wild-type tumors [28, 36, 68]. In the German Glioma Group retrospective study, *IDH* mutation influenced survival only in those patients who received radiation or chemotherapy immediately after surgery [24]. *IDH* mutation does not predict progression-free survival for temozolomide treatment in low grade astrocytomas that had previously received radiation [73]. *IDH* mutation may also predict the benefit of complete resection in high grade gliomas [4]. However, their retrospective nature and lack of control groups limits the conclusions that can be drawn from these studies.

MGMT, the gene encoding the DNA repair enzyme O6-methylguanine-DNA methyltransferase, is methylated in 30–40 % of GBMs and 80 % of *IDH*-mutated low grade gliomas [19, 27, 42]. The presence of methylated *MGMT* is prognostic in all grades of glioma, including both oligodendroglial and astrocytic histologies [42, 61, 70, 78]. Given the strong association between G-CIMP phenotype and *MGMT* methylation, the prognostic significance of each of these independently cannot be assessed. It is also not clear whether the observation that *MGMT* methylation is more significant than expression level measured by RNA or protein is due to biology or to technical artifacts of the assays used.

MGMT was originally studied because of its role in repairing damage from alkylating agents such as the nitrosoureas or temozolomide. However, it remains controversial whether *MGMT* methylation is predictive of benefit from temozolomide. In the long-term follow-up of EORTC 26981-22981/NCIC CE3, *MGMT* methylation was prognostic in both the radiation alone and radiation plus temozolomide groups. Moreover, there was a statistically significant improvement in survival with the addition of temozolomide in both the *MGMT* methylated and unmethylated groups with similar hazard ratio, although the absolute benefit was much smaller in the unmethylated group [70]. In the elderly population, two trials (NOA-08 and the Nordic trial) have suggested that people with GBM with *MGMT* methylation have improved survival with temozolomide monotherapy compared to radiation, while the opposite is true for elderly people with GBM with unmethylated *MGMT* [47, 85]. The role of *MGMT* or other potential biomarkers other than *IDH* in grade 2 or 3 astrocytomas remains uncertain.

7 Ependymomas

Ependymomas have been subtyped based on both location (supratentorial, infratentorial, or spinal cord) or by gene expression pattern. Common genetic alterations in ependymomas include *NF2* mutation or loss, *HER2/erbB2* and *erbB4* amplification, and *RASSF1A* and *HIC1* methylation [15, 20, 23, 81]. Two groups have used gene expression to identify two types of ependymoma, one characterized by growth factor receptor signaling and the other by large chromosomal rearrangements along with altered metabolism and cytoskeleton pathways [82, 86]. Most recently, a fusion gene involving c11orf95 and *relA*, the active component of NF-κB, was found to be a driver alteration in supratentorial ependymoma [52]. The high frequency observed of this fusion in the supratentorial ependymomas suggest that this is both a key driver of biology in this tumor subtype and may also be a potential target for specific drug development. Prognostic markers for ependymoma are not well established.

8 Conclusion

Gliomas include multiple distinct histopathologic types of tumors under the current WHO classification. Recent findings regarding some of the key driving alterations in some tumor types elucidate both the distinct biologies that define different histopathologies, and identify distinct molecular subtypes within single histopathologies. There appear to be at least three key molecular ontology pathways to the development of diffuse glioma. One pathway starts with *IDH* mutation followed by *TP53* mutation and results in astrocytic lineage tumors. These gliomas start as grade 2 astrocytomas, have the G-CIMP phenotype, and presumably then acquire other genetic alterations that result in progression to higher grade tumors. Another pathway starts with *IDH* mutation followed by loss of 1p/19q, which is associated with mutation in the *CIC* gene or the *FUBP1* gene. These alterations result in development of grade 2 oligodendrogliomas, which can then acquire other genetic alterations to become anaplastic oligodendrogliomas. The third pathway includes those gliomas that are wild-type for *IDH*. These gliomas appear to rapidly acquire multiple complex genetic alterations, including amplification or mutation of *EGFR*, and loss of the *PTEN* gene, and become GBMs very early in their development. *IDH*, 1p/19q codeletion, and *MGMT* are validated prognostic and probably predictive markers as well.

References

1. Alcantara Llaguno S, Chen J, Kwon CH, Jackson EL, Li Y, Burns DK, Alvarez-Buylla A, Parada LF (2009) Malignant astrocytomas originate from neural stem/progenitor cells in a somatic tumor suppressor mouse model. Cancer Cell 15(1):45–56. doi:10.1016/j.ccr.2008.12.006
2. Balss J, Meyer J, Mueller W, Korshunov A, Hartmann C, von Deimling A (2008) Analysis of the IDH1 codon 132 mutation in brain tumors. Acta Neuropathol 116(6):597–602. doi:10.1007/s00401-008-0455-2

3. Beier CP, Kumar P, Meyer K, Leukel P, Bruttel V, Aschenbrenner I, Riemenschneider MJ, Fragoulis A, Rummele P, Lamszus K, Schulz JB, Weis J, Bogdahn U, Wischhusen J, Hau P, Spang R, Beier D (2012) The cancer stem cell subtype determines immune infiltration of glioblastoma. Stem Cells Dev 21(15):2753–2761. doi:10.1089/scd.2011.0660
4. Beiko J, Suki D, Hess KR, Fox BD, Cheung V, Cabral M, Shonka N, Gilbert MR, Sawaya R, Prabhu SS, Weinberg J, Lang FF, Aldape KD, Sulman EP, Rao G, McCutcheon IE, Cahill DP (2014) IDH1 mutant malignant astrocytomas are more amenable to surgical resection and have a survival benefit associated with maximal surgical resection. Neuro-Oncology 16(1):81–91. doi:10.1093/neuonc/not159
5. Bettegowda C, Agrawal N, Jiao Y, Sausen M, Wood LD, Hruban RH, Rodriguez FJ, Cahill DP, McLendon R, Riggins G, Velculescu VE, Oba-Shinjo SM, Marie SK, Vogelstein B, Bigner D, Yan H, Papadopoulos N, Kinzler KW (2011) Mutations in CIC and FUBP1 contribute to human oligodendroglioma. Science 333(6048):1453–1455. doi:10.1126/science.1210557
6. Bhat KP, Balasubramaniyan V, Vaillant B, Ezhilarasan R, Hummelink K, Hollingsworth F, Wani K, Heathcock L, James JD, Goodman LD, Conroy S, Long L, Lelic N, Wang S, Gumin J, Raj D, Kodama Y, Raghunathan A, Olar A, Joshi K, Pelloski CE, Heimberger A, Kim SH, Cahill DP, Rao G, Den Dunnen WF, Boddeke HW, Phillips HS, Nakano I, Lang FF, Colman H, Sulman EP, Aldape K (2013) Mesenchymal differentiation mediated by NF-kappaB promotes radiation resistance in glioblastoma. Cancer Cell 24(3):331–346. doi:10.1016/j.ccr.2013.08.001
7. Bleeker FE, Lamba S, Leenstra S, Troost D, Hulsebos T, Vandertop WP, Frattini M, Molinari F, Knowles M, Cerrato A, Rodolfo M, Scarpa A, Felicioni L, Buttitta F, Malatesta S, Marchetti A, Bardelli A (2009) IDH1 mutations at residue p.R132 (IDH1(R132)) occur frequently in high-grade gliomas but not in other solid tumors. Hum Mutat 30(1):7–11. doi:10.1002/humu.20937
8. Brennan CW, Verhaak RG, McKenna A, Campos B, Noushmehr H, Salama SR, Zheng S, Chakravarty D, Sanborn JZ, Berman SH, Beroukhim R, Bernard B, Wu CJ, Genovese G, Shmulevich I, Barnholtz-Sloan J, Zou L, Vegesna R, Shukla SA, Ciriello G, Yung WK, Zhang W, Sougnez C, Mikkelsen T, Aldape K, Bigner DD, Van Meir EG, Prados M, Sloan A, Black KL, Eschbacher J, Finocchiaro G, Friedman W, Andrews DW, Guha A, Iacocca M, O'Neill BP, Foltz G, Myers J, Weisenberger DJ, Penny R, Kucherlapati R, Perou CM, Hayes DN, Gibbs R, Marra M, Mills GB, Lander E, Spellman P, Wilson R, Sander C, Weinstein J, Meyerson M, Gabriel S, Laird PW, Haussler D, Getz G, Chin L (2013) The somatic genomic landscape of glioblastoma. Cell 155(2):462–477. doi:10.1016/j.cell.2013.09.034
9. Cairncross G, Wang M, Shaw E, Jenkins R, Brachman D, Buckner J, Fink K, Souhami L, Laperriere N, Curran W, Mehta M (2013) Phase III trial of chemoradiotherapy for anaplastic oligodendroglioma: long-term results of RTOG 9402. J Clin Oncol: Official J Am Soc Clin Oncol 31(3):337–343. doi:10.1200/JCO.2012.43.2674
10. Chaudhry IH, O'Donovan DG, Brenchley PE, Reid H, Roberts IS (2001) Vascular endothelial growth factor expression correlates with tumour grade and vascularity in gliomas. Histopathol 39(4):409–415
11. Christensen BC, Smith AA, Zheng S, Koestler DC, Houseman EA, Marsit CJ, Wiemels JL, Nelson HH, Karagas MR, Wrensch MR, Kelsey KT, Wiencke JK (2011) DNA methylation, isocitrate dehydrogenase mutation, and survival in glioma. J Natl Cancer Inst 103(2):143–153. doi:10.1093/jnci/djq497
12. Cin H, Meyer C, Herr R, Janzarik WG, Lambert S, Jones DT, Jacob K, Benner A, Witt H, Remke M, Bender S, Falkenstein F, Van Anh TN, Olbrich H, von Deimling A, Pekrun A, Kulozik AE, Gnekow A, Scheurlen W, Witt O, Omran H, Jabado N, Collins VP, Brummer T, Marschalek R, Lichter P, Korshunov A, Pfister SM (2011) Oncogenic FAM131B-BRAF fusion resulting from 7q34 deletion comprises an alternative mechanism of MAPK pathway activation in pilocytic astrocytoma. Acta Neuropathol 121(6):763–774. doi:10.1007/s00401-011-0817-z
13. Dang L, White DW, Gross S, Bennett BD, Bittinger MA, Driggers EM, Fantin VR, Jang HG, Jin S, Keenan MC, Marks KM, Prins RM, Ward PS, Yen KE, Liau LM, Rabinowitz JD,

Cantley LC, Thompson CB, Vander Heiden MG, Su SM (2009) Cancer-associated IDH1 mutations produce 2-hydroxyglutarate. Nature 462(7274):739–744. doi:10.1038/nature08617
14. Dolecek T, Propp J, Stroup N, Kruchko C (2012) CBTRUS statistical report: primary brain and central nervous system tumors diagnosed in the United States in 2005–2009. Neuro-Oncology 15(suppl 5):1–49
15. Ebert C, von Haken M, Meyer-Puttlitz B, Wiestler OD, Reifenberger G, Pietsch T, von Deimling A (1999) Molecular genetic analysis of ependymal tumors. NF2 mutations and chromosome 22q loss occur preferentially in intramedullary spinal ependymomas. Am J Pathol 155(2):627–632. doi:10.1016/S0002-9440(10)65158-9
16. Figueroa ME, Abdel-Wahab O, Lu C, Ward PS, Patel J, Shih A, Li Y, Bhagwat N, Vasanthakumar A, Fernandez HF, Tallman MS, Sun Z, Wolniak K, Peeters JK, Liu W, Choe SE, Fantin VR, Paietta E, Lowenberg B, Licht JD, Godley LA, Delwel R, Valk PJ, Thompson CB, Levine RL, Melnick A (2010) Leukemic IDH1 and IDH2 mutations result in a hypermethylation phenotype, disrupt TET2 function, and impair hematopoietic differentiation. Cancer Cell 18(6):553–567. doi:10.1016/j.ccr.2010.11.015
17. Frattini V, Trifonov V, Chan JM, Castano A, Lia M, Abate F, Keir ST, Ji AX, Zoppoli P, Niola F, Danussi C, Dolgalev I, Porrati P, Pellegatta S, Heguy A, Gupta G, Pisapia DJ, Canoll P, Bruce JN, McLendon RE, Yan H, Aldape K, Finocchiaro G, Mikkelsen T, Prive GG, Bigner DD, Lasorella A, Rabadan R, Iavarone A (2013) The integrated landscape of driver genomic alterations in glioblastoma. Nat Genet 45(10):1141–1149. doi:10.1038/ng.2734
18. Garber K (2010) Oncometabolite? IDH1 discoveries raise possibility of new metabolism targets in brain cancers and leukemia. J Natl Cancer Inst 102(13):926–928. doi:10.1093/jnci/djq262
19. Gilbert MR, Wang M, Aldape KD, Stupp R, Hegi ME, Jaeckle KA, Armstrong TS, Wefel JS, Won M, Blumenthal DT, Mahajan A, Schultz CJ, Erridge S, Baumert B, Hopkins KI, Tzuk-Shina T, Brown PD, Chakravarti A, Curran WJ Jr, Mehta MP (2013) Dose-dense temozolomide for newly diagnosed glioblastoma: a randomized phase III clinical trial. J Clin Oncol: Official J American Society Clin Oncol 31(32):4085–4091. doi:10.1200/JCO.2013.49.6968
20. Gilbertson RJ, Bentley L, Hernan R, Junttila TT, Frank AJ, Haapasalo H, Connelly M, Wetmore C, Curran T, Elenius K, Ellison DW (2002) ERBB receptor signaling promotes ependymoma cell proliferation and represents a potential novel therapeutic target for this disease. Clin Cancer Res: An Official J American Assoc Cancer Res 8(10):3054–3064
21. Gronych J, Korshunov A, Bageritz J, Milde T, Jugold M, Hambardzumyan D, Remke M, Hartmann C, Witt H, Jones DT, Witt O, Heiland S, Bendszus M, Holland EC, Pfister S, Lichter P (2011) An activated mutant BRAF kinase domain is sufficient to induce pilocytic astrocytoma in mice. J Clin Investig 121(4):1344–1348. doi:10.1172/JCI44656
22. Hambardzumyan D, Cheng YK, Haeno H, Holland EC, Michor F (2011) The probable cell of origin of NF1- and PDGF-driven glioblastomas. PLoS ONE 6(9):24454. doi:10.1371/journal.pone.0024454
23. Hamilton DW, Lusher ME, Lindsey JC, Ellison DW, Clifford SC (2005) Epigenetic inactivation of the RASSF1A tumour suppressor gene in ependymoma. Cancer Lett 227 (1):75–81. doi:10.1016/j.canlet.2004.11.044
24. Hartmann C, Hentschel B, Tatagiba M, Schramm J, Schnell O, Seidel C, Stein R, Reifenberger G, Pietsch T, von Deimling A, Loeffler M, Weller M (2011) Molecular markers in low-grade gliomas: predictive or prognostic? Clin Cancer Res: An Official J American Assoc Cancer Res 17(13):4588–4599. doi:10.1158/1078-0432.CCR-10-3194
25. Hartmann C, Hentschel B, Wick W, Capper D, Felsberg J, Simon M, Westphal M, Schackert G, Meyermann R, Pietsch T, Reifenberger G, Weller M, Loeffler M, von Deimling A (2010) Patients with IDH1 wild type anaplastic astrocytomas exhibit worse prognosis than IDH1-mutated glioblastomas, and IDH1 mutation status accounts for the unfavorable prognostic effect of higher age: implications for classification of gliomas. Acta Neuropathol 120 (6):707–718. doi:10.1007/s00401-010-0781-z

26. Hartmann C, Meyer J, Balss J, Capper D, Mueller W, Christians A, Felsberg J, Wolter M, Mawrin C, Wick W, Weller M, Herold-Mende C, Unterberg A, Jeuken JW, Wesseling P, Reifenberger G, von Deimling A (2009) Type and frequency of IDH1 and IDH2 mutations are related to astrocytic and oligodendroglial differentiation and age: a study of 1,010 diffuse gliomas. Acta Neuropathol 118(4):469–474. doi:10.1007/s00401-009-0561-9
27. Hegi ME, Diserens AC, Gorlia T, Hamou MF, de Tribolet N, Weller M, Kros JM, Hainfellner JA, Mason W, Mariani L, Bromberg JE, Hau P, Mirimanoff RO, Cairncross JG, Janzer RC, Stupp R (2005) MGMT gene silencing and benefit from temozolomide in glioblastoma. The New England J Med 352(10):997–1003. doi:10.1056/NEJMoa043331
28. Houillier C, Wang X, Kaloshi G, Mokhtari K, Guillevin R, Laffaire J, Paris S, Boisselier B, Idbaih A, Laigle-Donadey F, Hoang-Xuan K, Sanson M, Delattre JY (2010) IDH1 or IDH2 mutations predict longer survival and response to temozolomide in low-grade gliomas. Neurology 75(17):1560–1566. doi:10.1212/WNL.0b013e3181f96282
29. Humphrey PA, Wong AJ, Vogelstein B, Zalutsky MR, Fuller GN, Archer GE, Friedman HS, Kwatra MM, Bigner SH, Bigner DD (1990) Anti-synthetic peptide antibody reacting at the fusion junction of deletion-mutant epidermal growth factor receptors in human glioblastoma. Proc Natl Acad Sci USA 87(11):4207–4211
30. Jiang H, Ren X, Cui X, Wang J, Jia W, Zhou Z, Lin S (2013) 1p/19q codeletion and IDH1/2 mutation identified a subtype of anaplastic oligoastrocytomas with prognosis as favorable as anaplastic oligodendrogliomas. Neuro-Oncology 15(6):775–782. doi:10.1093/neuonc/not027
31. Jiao Y, Killela PJ, Reitman ZJ, Rasheed AB, Heaphy CM, de Wilde RF, Rodriguez FJ, Rosemberg S, Oba-Shinjo SM, Nagahashi Marie SK, Bettegowda C, Agrawal N, Lipp E, Pirozzi C, Lopez G, He Y, Friedman H, Friedman AH, Riggins GJ, Holdhoff M, Burger P, McLendon R, Bigner DD, Vogelstein B, Meeker AK, Kinzler KW, Papadopoulos N, Diaz LA, Yan H (2012) Frequent ATRX, CIC, FUBP1 and IDH1 mutations refine the classification of malignant gliomas. Oncotarget 3(7):709–722
32. Jin G, Reitman ZJ, Spasojevic I, Batinic-Haberle I, Yang J, Schmidt-Kittler O, Bigner DD, Yan H (2011) 2-hydroxyglutarate production, but not dominant negative function, is conferred by glioma-derived NADP-dependent isocitrate dehydrogenase mutations. PLoS ONE 6(2): e16812. doi:10.1371/journal.pone.0016812
33. Jones DT, Kocialkowski S, Liu L, Pearson DM, Backlund LM, Ichimura K, Collins VP (2008) Tandem duplication producing a novel oncogenic BRAF fusion gene defines the majority of pilocytic astrocytomas. Cancer Res 68(21):8673–8677. doi:10.1158/0008-5472.CAN-08-2097
34. Jones DT, Kocialkowski S, Liu L, Pearson DM, Ichimura K, Collins VP (2009) Oncogenic RAF1 rearrangement and a novel BRAF mutation as alternatives to KIAA1549:BRAF fusion in activating the MAPK pathway in pilocytic astrocytoma. Oncogene 28(20):2119–2123. doi:10.1038/onc.2009.73
35. Jones PA, Baylin SB (2007) The epigenomics of cancer. Cell 128(4):683–692. doi:10.1016/j.cell.2007.01.029
36. Juratli TA, Kirsch M, Robel K, Soucek S, Geiger K, von Kummer R, Schackert G, Krex D (2012) IDH mutations as an early and consistent marker in low-grade astrocytomas WHO grade II and their consecutive secondary high-grade gliomas. J Neuro Oncol. doi:10.1007/s11060-012-0844-1
37. Kang MR, Kim MS, Oh JE, Kim YR, Song SY, Seo SI, Lee JY, Yoo NJ, Lee SH (2009) Mutational analysis of IDH1 codon 132 in glioblastomas and other common cancers. Int J cancer 125(2):353–355. doi:10.1002/ijc.24379
38. Keunen O, Johansson M, Oudin A, Sanzey M, Rahim SA, Fack F, Thorsen F, Taxt T, Bartos M, Jirik R, Miletic H, Wang J, Stieber D, Stuhr L, Moen I, Rygh CB, Bjerkvig R, Niclou SP (2011) Anti-VEGF treatment reduces blood supply and increases tumor cell invasion in glioblastoma. Proc Natl Acad Sci USA 108(9):3749–3754. doi:10.1073/pnas.1014480108
39. Kraus JA, Koopmann J, Kaskel P, Maintz D, Brandner S, Schramm J, Louis DN, Wiestler OD, von Deimling A (1995) Shared allelic losses on chromosomes 1p and 19q suggest a common origin of oligodendroglioma and oligoastrocytoma. J Neuropathol Exp Neurol 54(1):91–95

40. Laffaire J, Everhard S, Idbaih A, Criniere E, Marie Y, de Reynies A, Schiappa R, Mokhtari K, Hoang-Xuan K, Sanson M, Delattre JY, Thillet J, Ducray F (2011) Methylation profiling identifies 2 groups of gliomas according to their tumorigenesis. Neuro-Oncology 13(1):84–98. doi:10.1093/neuonc/noq110
41. Lai A, Kharbanda S, Pope WB, Tran A, Solis OE, Peale F, Forrest WF, Pujara K, Carrillo JA, Pandita A, Ellingson BM, Bowers CW, Soriano RH, Schmidt NO, Mohan S, Yong WH, Seshagiri S, Modrusan Z, Jiang Z, Aldape KD, Mischel PS, Liau LM, Escovedo CJ, Chen W, Nghiemphu PL, James CD, Prados MD, Westphal M, Lamszus K, Cloughesy T, Phillips HS (2011) Evidence for Sequenced Molecular Evolution of IDH1 Mutant Glioblastoma From a Distinct Cell of Origin. J Clin Oncol: Official J Am Soc Clin Oncol 29(34):4482–4490. doi:10.1200/JCO.2010.33.8715
42. Leu S, von Felten S, Frank S, Vassella E, Vajtai I, Taylor E, Schulz M, Hutter G, Hench J, Schucht P, Boulay JL, Mariani L (2013) IDH/MGMT-driven molecular classification of low-grade glioma is a strong predictor for long-term survival. Neuro-oncology 15(4):469–479. doi:10.1093/neuonc/nos317
43. Li Z, Bao S, Wu Q, Wang H, Eyler C, Sathornsumetee S, Shi Q, Cao Y, Lathia J, McLendon RE, Hjelmeland AB, Rich JN (2009) Hypoxia-inducible factors regulate tumorigenic capacity of glioma stem cells. Cancer Cell 15(6):501–513. doi:10.1016/j.ccr.2009.03.018
44. Liu C, Sage JC, Miller MR, Verhaak RG, Hippenmeyer S, Vogel H, Foreman O, Bronson RT, Nishiyama A, Luo L, Zong H (2011) Mosaic analysis with double markers reveals tumor cell of origin in glioma. Cell 146(2):209–221. doi:10.1016/j.cell.2011.06.014
45. Louis DN, Ohgaki H, Wiestler OD, Cavenee WK, Burger PC, Jouvet A, Scheithauer BW, Kleihues P (2007) The 2007 WHO classification of tumours of the central nervous system. Acta Neuropathol 114(2):97–109. doi:10.1007/s00401-007-0243-4
46. Lyden D, Hattori K, Dias S, Costa C, Blaikie P, Butros L, Chadburn A, Heissig B, Marks W, Witte L, Wu Y, Hicklin D, Zhu Z, Hackett NR, Crystal RG, Moore MA, Hajjar KA, Manova K, Benezra R, Rafii S (2001) Impaired recruitment of bone-marrow-derived endothelial and hematopoietic precursor cells blocks tumor angiogenesis and growth. Nat Med 7 (11):1194–1201. doi:10.1038/nm1101-1194
47. Malmstrom A, Gronberg BH, Marosi C, Stupp R, Frappaz D, Schultz H, Abacioglu U, Tavelin B, Lhermitte B, Hegi ME, Rosell J, Henriksson R (2012) Temozolomide versus standard 6-week radiotherapy versus hypofractionated radiotherapy in patients older than 60 years with glioblastoma: the Nordic randomised, phase 3 trial. Lancet Oncol 13(9):916–926. doi:10.1016/S1470-2045(12)70265-6
48. Mentlein R, Hattermann K, Held-Feindt J (2012) Lost in disruption: role of proteases in glioma invasion and progression. Biochim Biophys Acta 1825(2):178–185. doi:10.1016/j.bbcan.2011.12.001
49. Nakano I, Dougherty JD, Kim K, Klement I, Geschwind DH, Kornblum HI (2007) Phosphoserine phosphatase is expressed in the neural stem cell niche and regulates neural stem and progenitor cell proliferation. Stem Cells 25(8):1975–1984. doi:10.1634/stemcells.2007-0046
50. Noushmehr H, Weisenberger DJ, Diefes K, Phillips HS, Pujara K, Berman BP, Pan F, Pelloski CE, Sulman EP, Bhat KP, Verhaak RG, Hoadley KA, Hayes DN, Perou CM, Schmidt HK, Ding L, Wilson RK, Van Den Berg D, Shen H, Bengtsson H, Neuvial P, Cope LM, Buckley J, Herman JG, Baylin SB, Laird PW, Aldape K (2010) Identification of a CpG island methylator phenotype that defines a distinct subgroup of glioma. Cancer Cell 17(5):510–522. doi:10.1016/j.ccr.2010.03.017
51. Ohgaki H, Dessen P, Jourde B, Horstmann S, Nishikawa T, Di Patre PL, Burkhard C, Schuler D, Probst-Hensch NM, Maiorka PC, Baeza N, Pisani P, Yonekawa Y, Yasargil MG, Lutolf UM, Kleihues P (2004) Genetic pathways to glioblastoma: a population-based study. Cancer Res 64(19):6892–6899. doi:10.1158/0008-5472.CAN-04-1337
52. Parker M, Mohankumar KM, Punchihewa C, Weinlich R, Dalton JD, Li Y, Lee R, Tatevossian RG, Phoenix TN, Thiruvenkatam R, White E, Tang B, Orisme W, Gupta K, Rusch M, Chen X, Nagahawhatte P, Hedlund E, Finkelstein D, Wu G, Shurtleff S, Easton J, Boggs K, Yergeau

D, Vadodaria B, Mulder HL, Becksford J, Gupta P, Huether R, Ma J, Song G, Gajjar A, Merchant T, Boop F, Smith AA, Ding L, Lu C, Ochoa K, Zhao D, Fulton RS, Fulton LL, Mardis ER, Wilson RK, Downing JR, Green DR, Zhang J, Ellison DW, Gilbertson RJ (2014) C11orf95-RELA fusions drive oncogenic NF-kappaB signalling in ependymoma. Nature 506 (7489):451–455. doi:10.1038/nature13109
53. Parsons DW, Jones S, Zhang X, Lin JC, Leary RJ, Angenendt P, Mankoo P, Carter H, Siu IM, Gallia GL, Olivi A, McLendon R, Rasheed BA, Keir S, Nikolskaya T, Nikolsky Y, Busam DA, Tekleab H, Diaz LA Jr, Hartigan J, Smith DR, Strausberg RL, Marie SK, Shinjo SM, Yan H, Riggins GJ, Bigner DD, Karchin R, Papadopoulos N, Parmigiani G, Vogelstein B, Velculescu VE, Kinzler KW (2008) An integrated genomic analysis of human glioblastoma multiforme. Science 321(5897):1807–1812. doi:10.1126/science.1164382
54. Persson AI, Petritsch C, Swartling FJ, Itsara M, Sim FJ, Auvergne R, Goldenberg DD, Vandenberg SR, Nguyen KN, Yakovenko S, Ayers-Ringler J, Nishiyama A, Stallcup WB, Berger MS, Bergers G, McKnight TR, Goldman SA, Weiss WA (2010) Non-stem cell origin for oligodendroglioma. Cancer Cell 18(6):669–682. doi:10.1016/j.ccr.2010.10.033
55. Phillips HS, Kharbanda S, Chen R, Forrest WF, Soriano RH, Wu TD, Misra A, Nigro JM, Colman H, Soroceanu L, Williams PM, Modrusan Z, Feuerstein BG, Aldape K (2006) Molecular subclasses of high-grade glioma predict prognosis, delineate a pattern of disease progression, and resemble stages in neurogenesis. Cancer Cell 9(3):157–173. doi:10.1016/j.ccr.2006.02.019
56. Pietsch T, Valter MM, Wolf HK, von Deimling A, Huang HJ, Cavenee WK, Wiestler OD (1997) Expression and distribution of vascular endothelial growth factor protein in human brain tumors. Acta Neuropathol 93(2):109–117
57. Plate KH, Breier G, Weich HA, Risau W (1992) Vascular endothelial growth factor is a potential tumour angiogenesis factor in human gliomas in vivo. Nature 359(6398):845–848. doi:10.1038/359845a0
58. Raabe EH, Lim KS, Kim JM, Meeker A, Mao XG, Nikkhah G, Maciaczyk J, Kahlert U, Jain D, Bar E, Cohen KJ, Eberhart CG (2011) BRAF activation induces transformation and then senescence in human neural stem cells: a pilocytic astrocytoma model. Clin Cancer Res: An Official J American Assoc Cancer Res 17(11):3590–3599. doi:10.1158/1078-0432.CCR-10-3349
59. Reifenberger J, Reifenberger G, Liu L, James CD, Wechsler W, Collins VP (1994) Molecular genetic analysis of oligodendroglial tumors shows preferential allelic deletions on 19q and 1p. Am J Pathol 145(5):1175–1190
60. Reiss Y, Machein MR, Plate KH (2005) The role of angiopoietins during angiogenesis in gliomas. Brain Pathol 15(4):311–317
61. Sadones J, Michotte A, Veld P, Chaskis C, Sciot R, Menten J, Joossens EJ, Strauven T, D'Hondt LA, Sartenaer D, Califice SF, Bierau K, Svensson C, De Greve J, Neyns B (2009) MGMT promoter hypermethylation correlates with a survival benefit from temozolomide in patients with recurrent anaplastic astrocytoma but not glioblastoma. Eur J Cancer 45 (1):146–153. doi:10.1016/j.ejca.2008.09.002
62. Sanson M, Marie Y, Paris S, Idbaih A, Laffaire J, Ducray F, El Hallani S, Boisselier B, Mokhtari K, Hoang-Xuan K, Delattre JY (2009) Isocitrate dehydrogenase 1 codon 132 mutation is an important prognostic biomarker in gliomas. J clin Oncol: Official J Am Soc Clin Oncol 27(25):4150–4154 JCO.2009.21.9832[pii]/JCO.2009.21.9832
63. Sasaki M, Knobbe CB, Munger JC, Lind EF, Brenner D, Brustle A, Harris IS, Holmes R, Wakeham A, Haight J, You-Ten A, Li WY, Schalm S, Su SM, Virtanen C, Reifenberger G, Ohashi PS, Barber DL, Figueroa ME, Melnick A, Zuniga-Pflucker JC, Mak TW (2012) IDH1 (R132H) mutation increases murine haematopoietic progenitors and alters epigenetics. Nature. doi:10.1038/nature11323
64. Scherer H (1938) Structural development in gliomas. Am J Cancer 34:333–351
65. Scherer HJ (1940) A critical review: the pathology of cerebral gliomas. J Neurol Psychiatry 3 (2):147–177

66. Shaifer CA, Huang J, Lin PC (2010) Glioblastoma cells incorporate into tumor vasculature and contribute to vascular radioresistance. Int J Cancer 127(9):2063–2075. doi:10.1002/ijc.25249
67. Singh D, Chan JM, Zoppoli P, Niola F, Sullivan R, Castano A, Liu EM, Reichel J, Porrati P, Pellegatta S, Qiu K, Gao Z, Ceccarelli M, Riccardi R, Brat DJ, Guha A, Aldape K, Golfinos JG, Zagzag D, Mikkelsen T, Finocchiaro G, Lasorella A, Rabadan R, Iavarone A (2012) Transforming fusions of FGFR and TACC genes in human glioblastoma. Science 337 (6099):1231–1235. doi:10.1126/science.1220834
68. SongTao Q, Lei Y, Si G, YanQing D, HuiXia H, XueLin Z, LanXiao W, Fei Y (2012) IDH mutations predict longer survival and response to temozolomide in secondary glioblastoma. Cancer Sci 103(2):269–273. doi:10.1111/j.1349-7006.2011.02134.x
69. Sonoda Y, Kumabe T, Nakamura T, Saito R, Kanamori M, Yamashita Y, Suzuki H, Tominaga T (2009) Analysis of IDH1 and IDH2 mutations in Japanese glioma patients. Cancer Sci 100 (10):1996–1998 CAS1270 [pii] /j.1349-7006.2009.01270.x
70. Stupp R, Hegi ME, Mason WP, van den Bent MJ, Taphoorn MJ, Janzer RC, Ludwin SK, Allgeier A, Fisher B, Belanger K, Hau P, Brandes AA, Gijtenbeek J, Marosi C, Vecht CJ, Mokhtari K, Wesseling P, Villa S, Eisenhauer E, Gorlia T, Weller M, Lacombe D, Cairncross JG, Mirimanoff RO (2009) Effects of radiotherapy with concomitant and adjuvant temozolomide versus radiotherapy alone on survival in glioblastoma in a randomised phase III study: 5-year analysis of the EORTC-NCIC trial. Lancet Oncol 10(5):459–466. doi:10.1016/S1470-2045(09)70025-7
71. Sturm D, Witt H, Hovestadt V, Khuong-Quang DA, Jones DT, Konermann C, Pfaff E, Tonjes M, Sill M, Bender S, Kool M, Zapatka M, Becker N, Zucknick M, Hielscher T, Liu XY, Fontebasso AM, Ryzhova M, Albrecht S, Jacob K, Wolter M, Ebinger M, Schuhmann MU, van Meter T, Fruhwald MC, Hauch H, Pekrun A, Radlwimmer B, Niehues T, von Komorowski G, Durken M, Kulozik AE, Madden J, Donson A, Foreman NK, Drissi R, Fouladi M, Scheurlen W, von Deimling A, Monoranu C, Roggendorf W, Herold-Mende C, Unterberg A, Kramm CM, Felsberg J, Hartmann C, Wiestler B, Wick W, Milde T, Witt O, Lindroth AM, Schwartzentruber J, Faury D, Fleming A, Zakrzewska M, Liberski PP, Zakrzewski K, Hauser P, Garami M, Klekner A, Bognar L, Morrissy S, Cavalli F, Taylor MD, van Sluis P, Koster J, Versteeg R, Volckmann R, Mikkelsen T, Aldape K, Reifenberger G, Collins VP, Majewski J, Korshunov A, Lichter P, Plass C, Jabado N, Pfister SM (2012) Hotspot mutations in H3F3A and IDH1 define distinct epigenetic and biological subgroups of glioblastoma. Cancer Cell 22(4):425–437. doi:10.1016/j.ccr.2012.08.024
72. Sugiarto S, Persson AI, Munoz EG, Waldhuber M, Lamagna C, Andor N, Hanecker P, Ayers-Ringler J, Phillips J, Siu J, Lim DA, Vandenberg S, Stallcup W, Berger MS, Bergers G, Weiss WA, Petritsch C (2011) Asymmetry-defective oligodendrocyte progenitors are glioma precursors. Cancer Cell 20(3):328–340. doi:10.1016/j.ccr.2011.08.011
73. Taal W, Dubbink HJ, Zonnenberg CB, Zonnenberg BA, Postma TJ, Gijtenbeek JM, Boogerd W, Groenendijk FH, Kros JM, Kouwenhoven MC, van Marion R, van Heuvel I, van der Holt B, Bromberg JE, Sillevis Smitt PA, Dinjens WN, van den Bent MJ (2011) First-line temozolomide chemotherapy in progressive low-grade astrocytomas after radiotherapy: molecular characteristics in relation to response. Neuro-oncology 13(2):235–241. doi:10.1093/neuonc/noq177
74. Taylor MD, Poppleton H, Fuller C, Su X, Liu Y, Jensen P, Magdaleno S, Dalton J, Calabrese C, Board J, Macdonald T, Rutka J, Guha A, Gajjar A, Curran T, Gilbertson RJ (2005) Radial glia cells are candidate stem cells of ependymoma. Cancer Cell 8(4):323–335. doi:10.1016/j.ccr.2005.09.001
75. TCGA (2008) Comprehensive genomic characterization defines human glioblastoma genes and core pathways. Nature 455(7216):1061–1068. doi:10.1038/nature07385

76. van den Bent MJ, Brandes AA, Rampling R, Kouwenhoven MC, Kros JM, Carpentier AF, Clement PM, Frenay M, Campone M, Baurain JF, Armand JP, Taphoorn MJ, Tosoni A, Kletzl H, Klughammer B, Lacombe D, Gorlia T (2009) Randomized phase II trial of erlotinib versus temozolomide or carmustine in recurrent glioblastoma: EORTC brain tumor group study 26034. J Clin Oncol: Official J Am Soc Clin Oncol 27(8):1268–1274. doi:10.1200/JCO.2008.17.5984
77. van den Bent MJ, Brandes AA, Taphoorn MJ, Kros JM, Kouwenhoven MC, Delattre JY, Bernsen HJ, Frenay M, Tijssen CC, Grisold W, Sipos L, Enting RH, French PJ, Dinjens WN, Vecht CJ, Allgeier A, Lacombe D, Gorlia T, Hoang-Xuan K (2013) Adjuvant procarbazine, lomustine, and vincristine chemotherapy in newly diagnosed anaplastic oligodendroglioma: long-term follow-up of EORTC brain tumor group study 26951. J Clin Oncol: Official J Am Soc Clin Oncol 31(3):344–350. doi:10.1200/JCO.2012.43.2229
78. van den Bent MJ, Dubbink HJ, Sanson M, van der Lee-Haarloo CR, Hegi M, Jeuken JW, Ibdaih A, Brandes AA, Taphoorn MJ, Frenay M, Lacombe D, Gorlia T, Dinjens WN, Kros JM (2009) MGMT promoter methylation is prognostic but not predictive for outcome to adjuvant PCV chemotherapy in anaplastic oligodendroglial tumors: a report from EORTC Brain Tumor Group Study 26951. J Clin Oncol: Official J Am Soc Clin Oncol 27(35):5881–5886. doi:10.1200/JCO.2009.24.1034
79. Verhaak RG, Hoadley KA, Purdom E, Wang V, Qi Y, Wilkerson MD, Miller CR, Ding L, Golub T, Mesirov JP, Alexe G, Lawrence M, O'Kelly M, Tamayo P, Weir BA, Gabriel S, Winckler W, Gupta S, Jakkula L, Feiler HS, Hodgson JG, James CD, Sarkaria JN, Brennan C, Kahn A, Spellman PT, Wilson RK, Speed TP, Gray JW, Meyerson M, Getz G, Perou CM, Hayes DN (2010) Integrated genomic analysis identifies clinically relevant subtypes of glioblastoma characterized by abnormalities in PDGFRA, IDH1, EGFR, and NF1. Cancer Cell 17(1):98–110. doi:10.1016/j.ccr.2009.12.020
80. von Deimling A, von Ammon K, Schoenfeld D, Wiestler OD, Seizinger BR, Louis DN (1993) Subsets of glioblastoma multiforme defined by molecular genetic analysis. Brain Pathol 3 (1):19–26
81. Waha A, Koch A, Hartmann W, Mack H, Schramm J, Sorensen N, Berthold F, Wiestler OD, Pietsch T (2004) Analysis of HIC-1 methylation and transcription in human ependymomas. Int J Cancer 110(4):542–549. doi:10.1002/ijc.20165
82. Wani K, Armstrong TS, Vera-Bolanos E, Raghunathan A, Ellison D, Gilbertson R, Vaillant B, Goldman S, Packer RJ, Fouladi M, Pollack I, Mikkelsen T, Prados M, Omuro A, Soffietti R, Ledoux A, Wilson C, Long L, Gilbert MR, Aldape K (2012) A prognostic gene expression signature in infratentorial ependymoma. Acta Neuropathol 123(5):727–738. doi:10.1007/s00401-012-0941-4
83. Watanabe K, Tachibana O, Sata K, Yonekawa Y, Kleihues P, Ohgaki H (1996) Overexpression of the EGF receptor and p53 mutations are mutually exclusive in the evolution of primary and secondary glioblastomas. Brain Pathol 6(3):217–223 discussion 223-214
84. Watanabe T, Nobusawa S, Kleihues P, Ohgaki H (2009) IDH1 mutations are early events in the development of astrocytomas and oligodendrogliomas. Am J Pathol 174(4):1149–1153. doi:10.2353/ajpath.2009.080958
85. Wick W, Platten M, Meisner C, Felsberg J, Tabatabai G, Simon M, Nikkhah G, Papsdorf K, Steinbach JP, Sabel M, Combs SE, Vesper J, Braun C, Meixensberger J, Ketter R, Mayer-Steinacker R, Reifenberger G, Weller M (2012) Temozolomide chemotherapy alone versus radiotherapy alone for malignant astrocytoma in the elderly: the NOA-08 randomised, phase 3 trial. Lancet Oncol 13(7):707–715. doi:10.1016/S1470-2045(12)70164-X
86. Witt H, Mack SC, Ryzhova M, Bender S, Sill M, Isserlin R, Benner A, Hielscher T, Milde T, Remke M, Jones DT, Northcott PA, Garzia L, Bertrand KC, Wittmann A, Yao Y, Roberts SS, Massimi L, Van Meter T, Weiss WA, Gupta N, Grajkowska W, Lach B, Cho YJ, von Deimling A, Kulozik AE, Witt O, Bader GD, Hawkins CE, Tabori U, Guha A, Rutka JT, Lichter P, Korshunov A, Taylor MD, Pfister SM (2011) Delineation of two clinically and molecularly distinct subgroups of posterior fossa ependymoma. Cancer Cell 20(2):143–157. doi:10.1016/j.ccr.2011.07.007

87. Xu W, Yang H, Liu Y, Yang Y, Wang P, Kim SH, Ito S, Yang C, Xiao MT, Liu LX, Jiang WQ, Liu J, Zhang JY, Wang B, Frye S, Zhang Y, Xu YH, Lei QY, Guan KL, Zhao SM, Xiong Y (2011) Oncometabolite 2-hydroxyglutarate is a competitive inhibitor of alpha-ketoglutarate-dependent dioxygenases. Cancer Cell 19(1):17–30. doi:10.1016/j.ccr.2010.12.014
88. Yan H, Parsons DW, Jin G, McLendon R, Rasheed BA, Yuan W, Kos I, Batinic-Haberle I, Jones S, Riggins GJ, Friedman H, Friedman A, Reardon D, Herndon J, Kinzler KW, Velculescu VE, Vogelstein B, Bigner DD (2009) IDH1 and IDH2 mutations in gliomas. The New England journal of medicine 360(8):765–773. doi:10.1056/NEJMoa0808710
89. Yang B, Zhong C, Peng Y, Lai Z, Ding J (2010) Molecular mechanisms of "off-on switch" of activities of human IDH1 by tumor-associated mutation R132H. Cell Res 20(11):1188–1200. doi:10.1038/cr.2010.145
90. Zagzag D, Lukyanov Y, Lan L, Ali MA, Esencay M, Mendez O, Yee H, Voura EB, Newcomb EW (2006) Hypoxia-inducible factor 1 and VEGF upregulate CXCR4 in glioblastoma: implications for angiogenesis and glioma cell invasion. Lab Invest; J Tech Methods Pathol 86 (12):1221–1232. doi:10.1038/labinvest.3700482
91. Zhao J, Ma W, Zhao H (2014) Loss of heterozygosity 1p/19q and survival in glioma: a meta-analysis. Neuro-oncology 16(1):103–112. doi:10.1093/neuonc/not145
92. Zhao S, Guan KL (2010) IDH1 mutant structures reveal a mechanism of dominant inhibition. Cell Res 20(12):1279–1281. doi:10.1038/cr.2010.160
93. Zhao S, Lin Y, Xu W, Jiang W, Zha Z, Wang P, Yu W, Li Z, Gong L, Peng Y, Ding J, Lei Q, Guan KL, Xiong Y (2009) Glioma-derived mutations in IDH1 dominantly inhibit IDH1 catalytic activity and induce HIF-1alpha. Science 324(5924):261–265. doi:10.1126/science.1170944

Surgery for Gliomas

Matthew C. Tate

Abstract Surgical resection, with the goal of maximal tumor removal, is now standard of care for the overwhelming majority of newly diagnosed gliomas. In order to achieve this goal while minimizing the risk of postoperative neurologic deficits, intraoperative brain mapping remains the gold standard. Recent advances in technical aspects of preoperative and intraoperative brain mapping, as well as our understanding of the functional anatomy of the human brain with respect to language, movement, sensation, and cognition, particularly at the subcortical level, have improved our ability to safely perform aggressive resective surgeries in eloquent areas. In this chapter, the functional anatomy of the human brain relevant to intrinsic tumor resection is reviewed. In addition, general principles governing surgical management of patients are highlighted, with a particular emphasis on awake brain mapping.

Keywords Glioma surgery · Mapping

Contents

M.C. Tate (✉)
Department of Neurological Surgery, Northwestern University Feinberg School of Medicine, 676 North Saint Clair Street Suite 2210, 60611 Chicago, IL, USA
e-mail: matthew.tate@northwestern.edu

J. Raizer and A. Parsa (eds.), *Current Understanding and Treatment of Gliomas*,
Cancer Treatment and Research 163, DOI 10.1007/978-3-319-12048-5_3

1 Introduction

Recent data from multiple series have demonstrated the importance of aggressive surgical resection for improved outcomes in glioma. In particular, increased volumetric extent of resection has been shown to directly improve survival in both low-grade [1–5] and high-grade gliomas [6–9]. The mechanism of improved survival is likely by delaying malignant transformation in low-grade gliomas and similarly delaying progression in high-grade gliomas. Given the clear benefit of surgery, the primary goal of glioma surgery is to maximize the extent of resection while minimizing morbidity. Thus, it is imperative that neurosurgeons and neurooncologists have an understanding of the relevant cortical and subcortical functional networks, not only to plan and execute a surgical plan, but also to counsel patients with respect to risks and benefits of surgery. Despite advances in preoperative functional assessment in brain tumor patients, including functional MRI (fMRI), diffusion tensor imaging (DTI), magnetoencephalography (MEG), and transcranial magnetic stimulation (TMS), direct cortical stimulation (DCS) in the operating room remains the gold standard for identifying indispensable functional pathways to preserve function. In this chapter, the relevant cortical and subcortical functional anatomy in the human brain is reviewed, with a particular focus on data from intraoperative DCS. Basic principles guiding the preoperative evaluation, management, and surgical planning for patients with gliomas are discussed. Finally, a detailed description of surgical technique, including modern cortical/subcortical mapping protocols which allow for optimal surgical resection while minimizing neurologic deficits is provided.

2 Review of Human Cortical and Subcortical Functional Anatomy

2.1 Motor

Motor networks in the human cortex are primarily located within the frontal lobe. The primary motor cortex (M1) within the precentral gyrus, is bounded by the central sulcus posteriorly and the precentral sulcus anteriorly. DCS of M1 in

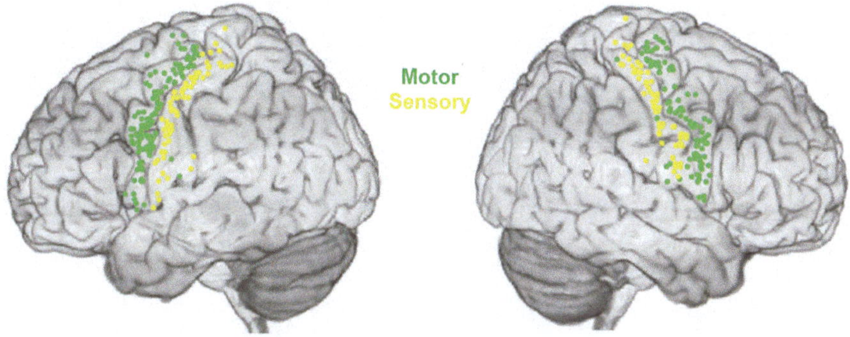

Fig. 1 Motor and sensory direct cortical stimulation data. Rendering of *left* and *right* hemisphere positive stimulation sites eliciting movement (*green*) and dysesthesias (*yellow*) within the precentral and postcentral gyri, respectively. Adapted from Tate et al. [41]

patients undergoing craniotomy reliably produces contralateral muscle contractions in a topographically organized fashion (Fig. 1). This phenomenon was first shown in humans by Sir Horsley in 1891 [10] and was followed by the demonstration of the motor homunculus by Penfield and Boldrey in 1937 [11]. At the subcortical level, DCS of M1 produces movement of a contralateral single muscle or limited group of muscles that is transmitted by the corticospinal tract (CST), and the patient is unable to suppress the movement. An exception to the general rule of contralateral contraction with M1 stimulation is that DCS within palate, pharynx, and tongue regions of M1 can cause bilateral muscle contractions.

In addition to the contribution of M1 to the CST, premotor and supplementary motor cortices anterior to M1 in the frontal lobe also contribute to the CST. The exact function of these so-called "higher-order" motor areas are less well understood, but recent studies have given some insight into their functional contributions. The premotor cortex (PMC), corresponding to Brodmann Area 6, is composed of a dorsal part (dPMC) that includes the posterior part of the superior and middle frontal gyri just anterior to the precentral sulcus, and a ventral part (vPMC) that is defined by the precentral gyrus from the Sylvian fissure to the level of the superior frontal sulcus. PMC lesions result in proximal muscle weakness and difficulty with sequencing of movements of the contralateral limb [12]. DCS of the vPMC in patients undergoing awake craniotomy for tumor resection reliably causes disorders of articulation [13], while DCS in the left hemisphere points to a role in language. The supplementary motor area (SMA), also a part of Brodmann area 6, is located in the medial/posterior portion of the superior frontal gyrus just anterior to leg motor cortex. The SMA is thought to be involved in motor planning, as SMA stimulation causes complex contralateral movements and resection of the SMA produces a stereotypical "SMA-syndrome" characterized by impairment of volitional movements, hemineglect, and dyspraxia of the contralateral limbs with preservation of muscle tone. If the SMA of the dominant (language) hemisphere is involved, difficulty initiating speech may also be observed. Deficits caused by SMA syndrome

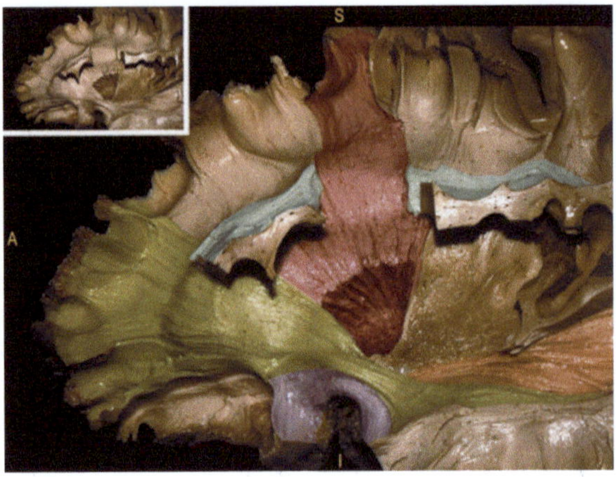

Fig. 2 Major white matter pathways. Dissected *left* hemisphere demonstrating main white matter pathways. Inferior frontal occipital fasciculus (IFOF, *green*); uncinated fasciculus (UF, *violet*); superior longitudinal fasciculus (SLF, *blue*); corticospinal tract (CST, *orange*). Inset shows colors prior to colorization. Adapted from De Benedictis et al. [42]

typically resolve within a few months postoperatively [14, 15]. As with M1, the SMA also demonstrates somatotopy: leg representation is most posterior, face is most anterior, and the arm region is located in between [14]. The frontal eye field (FEF) of the frontal lobe is located within the middle frontal gyrus just anterior to dPMC and is involved in saccadic eye movement. Lesions of the FEF impair voluntarily contralateral gaze, and DCS may elicit conjugate eye movements toward the contralateral side [16, 17].

In addition to motor regions located in the frontal lobe, the parietal lobe is involved in tuning of movement (preparation, control, adjustment). For example, the primary somatosensory area (S1), discussed further in the sensory section below, can produce complex motor movements when stimulated. Other proposed parietal lobe functions include visuomotor transformation and coding of motor acts such as grasping [18].

At the subcortical level, the major descending pathway is the corticospinal tract (CST) which originates as axons of pyramidal neurons within the layer V of M1 that travel through the centrum semiovale, corona radiata, posterior limb of the internal capsule, cerebral peduncle, pyramidal decussation in the medulla, and then descends as the lateral corticospinal spinal tract in the spinal cord (Fig. 2). The other major descending motor system is the corticobulbar tract, which originates in the cortical motor areas described above and descends alongside the corticospinal tracts before eventually projecting to brainstem motor cranial nerve nuclei bilaterally. The exception to this rule is innervation to the lower face, which is unilateral.

2.2 Sensory

The primary sensory pathway of relevance to glioma surgery is the posterior column–medial lemniscus pathway. Vibration, proprioceptive, and light touch sensory information from the periphery is detected by sensory neurons that have their cell body in the dorsal root ganglion and axon that ascends within the posterior column of the spinal cord and synapse onto ipsilateral gracile and cuneatus nuclei that are devoted to lower body and upper body sensation, respectively, within the caudal medulla. Second-order axons then cross the midline and ascend within the medial lemniscus within the contralateral brainstem and midbrain before eventually synapsing onto neurons of the ventral posterior lateral (VPL) nucleus of the thalamus. Neurons of the VPL then project to the layers III and IV of S1 [19]. S1 is within the postcentral gyrus of the parietal lobe, and electrical stimulation of S1 causes sensory perception, typically described as tingling (Fig. 1), in a localized region of the contralateral body, as initially described by Cushing in 1909 [20].

2.3 *Language*

2.3.1 Hemispheric Dominance

The concept of left hemispheric dominance for language was first proposed by Paul Broca in 1865 [21]. Current data are that for 85 % of the population the left hemisphere is dominant, while 9 % of patients have bilateral representation, and 6 % have right-sided dominance. For right-handed patients, 98 % have left-sided dominance. Thus, clinical investigation of dominance, the gold standard being the Wada test, is typically reserved for left-handed or ambidextrous patients. In addition to language, the left hemisphere is typically involved in logical problem solving and calculation. Conversely, the right hemisphere is specifically devoted to facial recognition, tasks involving visuospatial manipulation, and musicality [22].

2.3.2 Comprehension

Language comprehension was described by Wernicke as residing in the posterior superior temporal gyrus [23]. DCS studies have further expanded the region of language comprehension to include the posterior portion of both the superior and middle temporal gyri, as well as the inferior parietal lobule superior to the Sylvian fissure. Damage to any of these areas can result in a receptive aphasia, in which the patient can still produce written or oral language with normal grammar/syntax/prosody, but the word content is incorrect, often with neologisms or word salad. In addition, the ability to repeat words and name pictures is compromised, although naming and language comprehension may be mediated by distinct regions of the posterior superior temporal lobe [24]. In addition, the ability to sing and to recite memorized passages is maintained. If similar areas are damaged in the nondominant hemisphere, dysprosody may occur, which is the inability to detect the pitch, rhythm, or emotional content of speech. More recent studies have aimed to further dissect various aspects of language within the parietal-temporal-occipital junction. From these studies, we have learned that the posterior temporal lobe is involved in reading and word retrieval but not particularly involved in word repetition.

2.3.3 Language Output

Classically, the final common pathway of language output is known as Broca's area, which encompasses the pars triangularis and pars opercularis within the posterior third of the inferior frontal gyrus. However, recent studies point to the ventral dPMC as the final common speech output region, while Broca's area may be more involved in higher order speech processing. Thus, stimulation of vPMC typically causes overt speech arrest, while stimulation at Broca's area causes dysnomias. Interestingly, the inferior frontal gyrus of the nondominant hemisphere appears to be involved in the speech prosody (rhythm/stress/intonation of speech), with lesions to this area causing flat, unemotional speech [25]. In addition, as mentioned earlier in the chapter, the SMA of the dominant hemisphere is involved in speech initiation, and stimulation can cause temporary speech arrest or vocalization. Finally, the dominant insular cortex may plan an important role in speech planning [26].

Recent insights from cortical stimulation studies have refined our understanding of the relationship of writing. While circuits involved in writing do correspond to the same hemisphere as oral language, at least some of the writing sites are partially distinct, as evidenced by the presence of writing deficits despite negative mapping at traditional language sites. Areas shown to be important for writing function include the dominant hemisphere superior parietal lobe, supramarginal gyrus, insula, middle and inferior frontal gyri, and SMA [27].

2.3.4 Subcortical Language Representation

The major subcortical pathways subserving oral language function as identified by direct intraoperative stimulation are the superior longitudinal fasciculus (SLF) and inferior occipito-frontal fasciculus (Fig. 2). The SLF connects the parietal/temporal region with the frontal lobe and is composed of two functionally distinct white matter pathways—the arcuate fasciculus (AF) and an indirect pathway parallel and lateral to the AF termed the lateral SLF (latSLF). The AF (also termed the dorsal phonologic stream) connects the posterior middle and inferior frontal gyri with the posterior portion of the middle and inferior temporal gyri, with interruption at any site along the pathway resulting in phonological disturbances. The latSLF, which connects the posterior superior temporal gyrus, supramarginal gyrus, and primarily vPMC, is involved in speech perception and articulation. The inferior frontal occipital fasciculus, also termed the ventral semantic stream, is involved with semantic aspects of speech and stimulation of the pathway intraoperatively produces semantic paraphasias. Finally, the subcallosal fasciculus, connecting the mesial frontal lobe structures (SMA, cingulate) to the caudate nucleus may mediate the control of language, with lesions resulting in transcortical motor aphasias characterized by nonfluent aphasia with intact repetition.

A number of studies have investigated the representation of languages in multilingual patients. A consistent finding is that both shared and language-specific sites are present in bilingual patients. While primary language and shared language sites are found throughout the temporal, parietal, and frontal lobes, distinct secondary language sites are located in the posterior temporal and parietal regions [28]. Interestingly, a recent study using DCS in bilingual patients implicate the dominant posterior temporal area and SLF in mediating language switching [29].

2.4 Vision

Visual information enters the retina and is transmitted via axons of retinal ganglion cells in the optic nerves, which cross at the optic chiasm and continue as the optic tracts which synapse in the lateral geniculate nucleus (LGN) of the thalamus. Cells of the LGN then project to the primary visual cortex of the occipital lobe via a fan-like projection of fibers (optic radiations) that pass lateral and superior to the atria and temporal horn of the lateral ventricle. The inferior optic radiations (Meyer's loop) project through the temporal lobe, carrying visual information from the contralateral superior visual field, with lesions causing a "pie in the sky" contralateral homonymous superior quadrantanopsia, though the ipsilateral eye is typically affected to a greater extent because of the lateral position of ipsilateral relative to contralateral eye fibers in the optic radiations [19]. Superior optic radiations project through the inferior parietal lobe and carry visual information from the contralateral inferior quadrants. The primary visual cortex resides in the occipital lobe along both borders of the calcarine sulcus and is retinotopically organized.

2.5 Spatial Cognition

The nondominant parietal lobe has been implicated in visuospatial perception, with damage to this region in humans producing a clinical syndrome of unilateral neglect, where patients essentially ignore the left half of their visual field. Recent studies using a line bisection task in awake human patients undergoing DCS has further defined the regions responsible for spatial cognition as both the supramarginal gyrus and posterior superior temporal lobe of the nondominant hemisphere [30]. Subcortically, both the optic radiations and nondominant SLF are involved in visuospatial information transmission.

3 Tumor Location and Extraoperative Assessment of Functional Regions

3.1 Tumor Imaging

Preoperative image of patients harboring gliomas begin with standard MRI sequences, most importantly T1-weighted images with gadolinium and T2/FLAIR.

In addition to providing anatomic localization of the tumor, the presence of enhancing tumor presents a target for surgical resection, as tumor recurrence risk is greatest within 2 cm of the enhancing rim [31]. Also, enhancement generally indicates the presence of a high-grade tumor, although there are exceptions. FLAIR sequences demonstrate the extent of edema, although one cannot determine the relative contributions of tumor versus vasogenic edema. With that caveat, for the case of low-grade gliomas (LGG), FLAIR signal is generally considered the target of resection. MR spectroscopy may be a useful adjunct in the setting of previously treated patients for which the diagnosis of recurrence versus treatment effect is equivocal.

3.2 Identifying Functional Brain Regions

3.2.1 Anatomic Localization of Functional Regions with MRI and DTI

In order to determine the relationship of the tumor to the Rolandic (sensorimotor) cortices, it is imperative that the surgeon be able to localize the central sulcus from preoperative MRI. Multiple methods exist for identifying the central sulcus (CS). On high-vertex axial images, mirror-image transverse sulci that are nearly perpendicular to the midline represent the CS (Fig. 3). The "hand knob", an omega-shaped region of the precentral gyrus, can usually be seen anterior to the CS. Another method is to analyze a sagittal MRI image at the midline. The cingulate sulcus is identified and

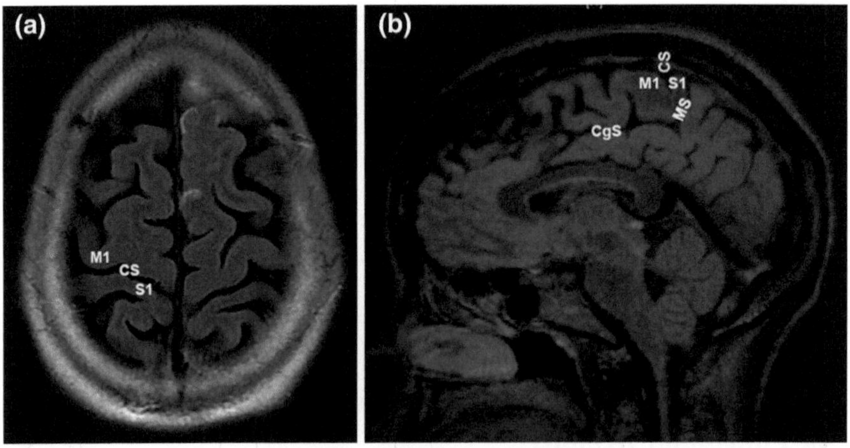

Fig. 3 Primary motor and sensory cortex landmarks on MRI. **a** Axial plane cut near the vertex illustrating hand knob within primary motor area (*M1*) of precentral gyrus and primary sensory area (*S1*) of postcentral gyrus anterior and posterior to central sulcus (*CS*), respectively. **b** Sagittal MRI slice just off *midline* showing paracentral lobule containing *M1*, *S1*, and *CS*. In this view, the cingulate sulcus (*CgS*) at its posterior extent angles superiorly to form the marginal sulcus (*MS*), which is continuous with the postcentral sulcus that forms the posterior border of *S1*

followed posteriorly and then superiorly where it terminates as the marginal sulcus. Immediately anterior to the marginal sulcus is the paracentral lobule, which is a medial extension of both the precentral (motor) and postcentral gyri of the lateral hemisphere. A third method utilizes a sagittal MRI image through the superficial portion of the inferior frontal gyrus, where pars triangularis and pars opercularis are identified. The vPMC is located just posterior to the precentral sulcus, and just posterior to vPMC is the inferior portion of the postcentral gyrus.

In addition to these topographic assessments of sensorimotor function, diffusion tensor imaging (DTI) is emerging as a routine part of preoperative evaluation of brain tumor patients as well as an important intraoperative adjunct to DCS. DTI fundamentally measures the degree of water diffusion within brain compartments, with more anisotropic regions such as white matter tracts having restricted directionality. The diffusion tensor can be evaluated for each MRI voxel of interest and a three-dimensional map is generated which accurately displays major white matter bundles, such as the CST, AF, SLF, IFOF, ILF, optic radiations, corpus callosum, and cingulum. While the process is associated with some inherent error and must be verified with direct stimulation in the operating room, in our experience DTI is helpful in determining the mapping strategy for a given tumor, discussing expectations with patients, and improving the efficiency of mapping in the operative room. As a general rule, DTI maps tend to be larger than that observed by direct stimulation, suggesting that resection of a significant part of a DTI-defined tract can be well tolerated in terms of maintaining function and highlighting the importance of direct stimulation during resection.

In contrast to preoperative localization of cortical and subcortical motor function, for which the standard MRI, DTI, and fMRI findings are relatively consistent between patients, functional language circuits are more diffuse and variable, making anatomic localization preoperatively more difficult. One particularly promising strategy is the use of preoperative DTI to localize language circuits. Recent data from a series of 230 patients undergoing glioma resection for whom the concordance of preoperative DTI with direct subcortical stimulation during surgery demonstrated a high concordance rate for the CST (motor), SLF (phonemic language), and frontal occipital fasciculus (semantic language) [32]. Thus, DTI is becoming an important preoperative and intraoperative adjunct to direct cortical mapping.

3.2.2 Functional Magnetic Resonance Imaging (fMRI)

fMRI is based on the principle that neurons of more active brain regions receive increased blood flow, which results in a localized increase of oxyhemoglobin (diamagnetic) relative to deoxyhemoglobin (paramagnetic). While localization of primary motor and sensory cortices by fMRI is accurate, several issues plague its widespread clinical use in brain tumor patients. First, at its most basic level, fMRI only demonstrates areas of increased blood flow, which is an indirect measure of neuronal activity. Also, the time lag between neuronal firing and diverted blood flow may be problematic for interpretation, particularly for complex actions involving several brain regions or which have overlapping neural circuitry, such as language or higher order cognitive function. fMRI at best illustrates which brain regions are involved in a particular task, but it does not indicate which regions are functionally necessary.

3.2.3 Magnetoencephalography (MEG)

Another methodology for detecting recruited neural circuitry during a given activity is MEG. Unlike fMRI, MEG directly measures the magnetic field produced by electrical activity in the brain, specifically dendritic potentials. During a particular task, changes in the magnitude of α, β, and γ band cerebral oscillations can be detected, with higher and lower frequencies representing synchronization and re-synchronization, respectively [33]. For example, changes in the γ frequency band are associated with higher order cognitive processes such as language processing [34]. MSI, which refers to incorporating MEG-based functional data into intraoperative brain navigation software, is being utilized in some centers. A recent study demonstrated a 100 % negative predictive value and 64 % positive predictive value for correlation of intraoperative stimulation of functional sites with MEG [35]. Thus, MEG presents a promising technology for identifying function or absence of function near the tumor preoperatively, although additional validation with DCS and outcome data will be necessary before routine use is recommended.

3.2.4 Transcranial Magnetic Stimulation (TMS)

A more recent technology for mapping cortical function preoperatively is TMS. TMS is a noninvasive technique that generates a precise, local magnetic field that induces an action potential in a small population of neurons. In the outpatient setting, through a simple algorithm the patient's MRI data can be coregistered with the TMS software, allowing for precise delivery of the magnetic field to the cortical surface. A magnetic field is delivered to specific regions of the primary motor cortex using the MRI-based map, resulting in pyramidal neuron activation and subsequent movements of the relevant contralateral muscle groups, which can then be detected by EMG. Recent data indicate that TMS-based motor maps correlate well with DCS in the operating room [36]. TMS has also been investigated as preoperative test for localization of language functions, though these data are somewhat less consistent compared to motor mapping [37]. Nonetheless, TMS represents a very promising modality not only for preoperative mapping of various cerebral functions but also a tool to study cortical plasticity before and after tumor resection, an important consideration for surgical strategies following initial resection.

4 Preoperative Considerations

After initial imaging studies to evaluate the tumor characteristics location and its location to known functional pathways and a careful neurological examination, it is important to consider the goals of surgery. For patients with diffuse disease, poor performance status, or for tumors located in the basal ganglia, thalamus, or brainstem, a biopsy to establish diagnosis may be the most prudent course of action. For a patient with a tumor within the primary motor cortex that has imaging characteristics of a low-grade glioma and minimal or no functional deficit, observation with frequent serial MRI scans is reasonable, based on the concept that additional functional pathways may be recruited over time. In these patients, a worsening neurologic deficit or evidence of progression would be criteria for operative intervention. Otherwise, craniotomy with the goal of maximal resection while minimizing morbidity is typically the first course of action. Once the decision is made to proceed with resection, the next major decision is whether the patient needs direct cortical mapping. Given the broad distribution of functional areas in the human brain, the variation of function between patients, and the diffuse nature of intrinsic brain tumors, direct cortical and subcortical stimulation mapping can be justified for any intrinsic tumor, independent of hemisphere. At a minimum, tumors in the following regions require direct mapping, as they involve motor, sensory, or language areas: bilateral precentral and postcentral gyri, left middle/posterior temporal lobe, left inferior parietal lobule, and middle/posterior left superior/middle/inferior frontal gyri. With the exception of motor mapping, which can be performed with the patient under general anesthesia, these surgeries are performed under awake conditions. It is our tradition to also perform motor mapping in the awake state, as the efficiency and fidelity of the motor map are improved with the patient under local anesthesia. Patients with less than antigravity strength (0–2/5) or with significant preoperative language deficits (>25 % error rate) that do not improve with short-course steroids may not be good candidates for mapping. Also pediatric patients or more generally patients who may not be able to cooperate with the intraoperative tasks should not be offered awake craniotomy. For these scenarios, the approach would be able to perform either asleep mapping (for tumors in/near motor cortex) or to perform a more conservative resection based on anatomic imaging and available preoperative functional data. Finally, for the subset of patients with preoperative breakthrough seizures despite adequate anticonvulsant trials, electrocorticography can be used to guide resection of seizure foci in addition to the planned tumor resection. Such electrocorticography-guided glioma resections are particularly effective in reducing long-term seizure profiles in the pediatric population [38].

5 Intraoperative Mapping Techniques

5.1 Patient Positioning and Incision

The main considerations for positioning the patient in the operating room are related to the location of the tumor. A recent paper by Berger and Hadjipanayis [16] provides an excellent review of patient positioning and suggested skin incision as a function of tumor location. After appropriate positioning, all pressure points are padded. Importantly, the contralateral body must remain free of lines, blood pressure cuff, etc., so that it can be readily visualized during mapping. A heating blanket is placed to ensure temperature >36 °C. Intravenous steroids (4 mg decadron) and preoperative antibiotics (1–2 g cefazolin) are administered. Anticonvulsants are also administered, either the patient's home regimen or a dilantin load (15 mg/kg) if not previously on anticonvulsants. If elevated intracranial pressure is a concern, mannitol (1 g/kg) can be administered. Finally, a time-out procedure verifying patient characteristics, tumor side, surgical plan, expected blood loss, and details of the proposed mapping strategy is essential.

5.2 Awake Craniotomy

Ultimately, the success of awake craniotomy and language mapping relies on a cooperative patient. Given that the length of surgery may be several hours, it is important to have the patient comfortably sedated for the portions of the operation when mapping is not performed. While there are multiple options, a combination of propofol (≤100 μg/kg/min) and remifentanil (≥0.05 μg/kg/min) is common. It is important to ensure adequate ventilation and thus not to over sedate. For mild obstruction, a nasal airway can be helpful. Propofol is administered at the time of foley administration and just prior to Mayfield pin application. Lidocaine/bupivacaine local anesthetic is also administered at the three pin sites. Specifically, the local block should address the territories of the supraorbital (above midpoint of orbital rim), auriculotemporal (1.5 cm anterior to tragus), zygomaticotemporal (midway between supraorbital ridge and the posterior margin of the zygoma), and lesser/greater occipital nerves (along line extending from inion to mastoid), depending on the location of the anterior–posterior extent of the scalp incision. The propofol/remifentanil infusion is titrated during incision, muscle dissection, and craniotomy so that the patient remains comfortably sedated and breathing comfortably. After the bone flap is removed, all sedatives are discontinued and the patient is allowed to wake fully prior to opening the dura, as emergence can otherwise cause coughing and brain herniation, particularly for tumors with significant mass effect/edema. In addition, a 30-gauge needle is used to administer local to the dura along the middle meningeal artery. During mapping, propofol should be within six inches of the IV line and ice cold lactated Ringer's solution should be available should seizures occur during stimulation. Following mapping, propofol/remifentanil infusions are used to slowly increase the level of sedation while avoiding respiratory depression.

5.3 Asleep Craniotomy

The patient is premedicated with midazolam and then brought to the operating room. Induction is performed using fentanyl and propofol. The patient is paralyzed prior to intubation and the blockade is reversed following skin incision. General anesthesia is maintained with nitrous oxide (70 %), low-dose inhalational agent (typically <0.5 MAC isoflurane), and a fentanyl infusion (2 μg/kg/hr). After bone flap removal, mannitol and/or hyperventilation can be utilized if the brain appears full. Prior to initiation of motor mapping, the contralateral arm and leg should be uncovered and adequate patient temperature (>36 °C), and full reversal of neuromuscular blockade should be confirmed. As with awake mapping, first cold saline and then propofol can be used to abort seizure activity during mapping. Following completion of motor mapping, neuromuscular blockade can be resumed and is not reversed until after Mayfield pin removal. Fentanyl infusion is continued through scalp closure.

5.4 Mapping Details

5.4.1 Sensory/Motor Mapping

Following dural opening, an Ojemann Cortical Stimulator (biphasic square wave, 60 Hz, 1 ms duration, current range 2–16 mA peak–peak) is brought into the field for motor mapping. Stimulation is performed by applying a bipolar electrode to the cortical surface for 2 s. For asleep motor mapping, a starting current of 4 mA (peak–peak) is applied the primary motor cortex (as localized on MRI as discussed above), and the current increased in intervals of 2 mA until either an overt motor response or reproducible EMG activity in the muscle is noted. This latter EMG-based method is more sensitive than muscle contraction, allowing for decreased stimulation threshold and thus decreased risk of intraoperative seizure activity [39]. Positive cortical sites are labeled with sterile numbered paper squares and/or captured and saved onto the patient's navigated MRI sequence. Typically, motor stimulation is elicited in the face or hand region of the motor strip. Following mapping of the primary motor area, sensory mapping may be performed within the postcentral gyrus at the same current intensity, with patients typically reporting dysesthesias. Respecting the positive motor and sensory sites, cortical window(s) are opened to provide adequate access to the intrinsic tumor below the surface. Subcortical motor mapping is performed once the resection nears the CST system descending corticospinal fibers, internal capsule, cerebral peduncle. Prior to dural closure, a final stimulation at the cortical surface with preserved EMG activity distally provides confidence to the surgeon that the entire motor circuit is intact, whether subcortical stimulation was positive or not. Thus, even in the presence of a new postoperative motor deficit, the patient can be reassured that function will likely return.

5.4.2 Awake Language Mapping

For patients undergoing awake language mapping, all sedation is discontinued prior to dural opening. After the dura is opened and prior to mapping, orientation and counting are checked to ensure a baseline level of patient function and cooperation. The motor pathways are identified as described for asleep motor mapping, with the exception that stimulation is started at a lower current (1 mA) and increased in intervals of 0.5 mA. Language mapping begins a simple counting paradigm to investigate sites of speech arrest (typically within vPMC). Next, a picture naming task is employed where the patient looks at a computer screen and identifies simple objects presented at 4 s intervals. All sources of extraneous noise (suction tubing, pulse oximeter volume, etc.) are reduced to a minimum, and the patient is equipped with a microphone to ensure that the surgical team can hear all responses. The ability of the patient to correctly perform the task is verified prior to intratask stimulation to ensure that the sedation is adequately reversed and that there are no anesthesia-related changes from baseline language function. It may be necessary to adjust the draping, increase the time interval between picture refreshing, or adjust the patient's microphone setting to optimize patient comfort/cooperation and mapping efficiency. Once reliable picture naming is established, cortical stimulation is performed at 1 cm spacing throughout the exposed cortex. Stimulation is performed just prior to a picture change, and each stimulation-accompanied picture change is followed by one without stimulation to allow for recovery to baseline if an error is made and to serve as an internal control. A site is considered positive if stimulation-induced errors were present for at least 2 out of 3 trials. For each picture, the patient is asked to state "This is a …." followed by the object name, to enable the surgeon to distinguish speech arrest from anomia. After picture naming is complete, a similar stimulation paradigm is employed as the patient is asked to read a series of words presented on the computer screen, and sites with stimulation-induced alexia/dyslexia are recorded. For multilingual patients, given that some representation of each language is distinct, it is important to map each language separately, starting with the patient's primary language [28]. After localizing cortical representation of language, a corticectomy is planned utilizing these patient-specific functional data. During tumor resection, frequent subcortical stimulation, in conjunction with DTI tracts incorporated within the MRI-based navigation software and more importantly the surgeon's three-dimensional knowledge white matter anatomy, allows for reliable identification of the major language tracts, particularly the SLF/AF and IFOF. Subcortical stimulation of the SLF, AF, and IFOF at any part of the pathway reproducibly elicits dysarthria, phonemic paraphasias, and semantic paraphasias, respectively. In addition to these awake mapping techniques, the patient is asked to perform relevant functional tasks continuously throughout the resection as a method of functional monitoring.

6 Neural Plasticity: Implications for Surgical Management of Gliomas

Given the increasing evidence for redistribution of neural function in patients harboring gliomas, particularly in the case of low-grade gliomas (LGG), taking advantage of this property is becoming an important aspect of tumor management. For example, patients with LGG in the primary motor cortex may be observed over some period of time to allow for unmasking of latent or parallel circuits so that when resection becomes mandatory due to tumor growth or worsened neurologic function, the primary motor circuits are farther away from the tumor center. More recently, a number of groups have endorsed a strategy pioneered by Duffau which takes advantage of surgery-induced plasticity for LGG [40]. For patients with a limited first resection due to positive mapping findings within the planned resection field, the patient is allowed to recover and functional mapping is continued post-operatively via fMRI. Over the course of a few years, the eloquent function redistributes, presumably triggered by the initial surgery and/or long-standing slowly progressive tumor infiltration. Thus, at a second surgery the cortical area once devoted to a functional pathway which has been redistributed can be safely resected after proper confirmation of this functional shift with DCS. Importantly, this functional plasticity allowing for a more complete resection can occur over a relatively short time period relative to the expected time scale of tumor transformation to a higher grade.

7 Conclusions

The goal of modern glioma surgery is to maximize extent of resection while minimizing neurologic deficits. For patients with tumors in or near eloquent brain regions, DCS during resection allows for accurate localization of functional circuits at both the cortical and subcortical levels, including motor, sensory, language, vision, and spatial attention. In addition to direct cortical/subcortical stimulation, recent advances in preoperative mapping techniques such as fMRI, magnetoencephalography, diffusion tensor imaging, and TMS allow neurosurgeons to tailor respective strategies based on an individual patient's occupation, goals, and hobbies, thereby achieving not only the oncologic goals of maximal resection but also allowing the patient to return to normal life postoperatively.

References

1. Capelle L et al (2013) Spontaneous and therapeutic prognostic factors in adult hemispheric World Health Organization Grade II gliomas: a series of 1097 cases: clinical article. J Neurosurg 118(6):1157–1168
2. Claus EB et al (2005) Survival rates in patients with low-grade glioma after intraoperative magnetic resonance image guidance. Cancer 103(6):1227–1233
3. Jakola AS et al (2012) Comparison of a strategy favoring early surgical resection vs a strategy favoring watchful waiting in low-grade gliomas. JAMA 308(18):1881–1888
4. Smith JS et al (2008) Role of extent of resection in the long-term outcome of low-grade hemispheric gliomas. J Clin Oncol 26(8):1338–1345
5. van Veelen ML et al (1998) Supratentorial low grade astrocytoma: prognostic factors, dedifferentiation, and the issue of early versus late surgery. J Neurol Neurosurg Psychiatry 64 (5):581–587
6. Keles GE, Anderson B, Berger MS (1999) The effect of extent of resection on time to tumor progression and survival in patients with glioblastoma multiforme of the cerebral hemisphere. Surg Neurol 52(4):371–379
7. Lacroix M et al (2001) A multivariate analysis of 416 patients with glioblastoma multiforme: prognosis, extent of resection, and survival. J Neurosurg 95(2):190–198
8. Sanai N et al (2011) An extent of resection threshold for newly diagnosed glioblastomas. J Neurosurg 115(1):3–8
9. Stummer W et al (2006) Fluorescence-guided surgery with 5-aminolevulinic acid for resection of malignant glioma: a randomised controlled multicentre phase III trial. Lancet Oncol 7 (5):392–401
10. Horsley V (1891) The Croonian Lecture: on the mammalian nervous system, its funcitions and their localization, determined by an electrical method. Philos Trans Royal Soc London 82:60
11. Penfield W, Boldrey E (1937) Somatic motor and sensory representation in the cerebral cortex of man as studied by electrical stimulation. Brain 60:55
12. Freund HJ, Hummelsheim H (1985) Lesions of premotor cortex in man. Brain 108(Pt 3):697–733
13. Duffau H et al (2003) The role of dominant premotor cortex in language: a study using intraoperative functional mapping in awake patients. Neuroimage 20(4):1903–1914
14. Fontaine D, Capelle L, Duffau H (2002) Somatotopy of the supplementary motor area: evidence from correlation of the extent of surgical resection with the clinical patterns of deficit. Neurosurgery 50(2):297–303 (discussion 303–305)
15. Rostomily RC et al (1991) Postoperative deficits and functional recovery following removal of tumors involving the dominant hemisphere supplementary motor area. J Neurosurg 75 (1):62–68
16. Berger MS, Hadjipanayis CG (2007) Surgery of intrinsic cerebral tumors. Neurosurgery 61(1 Suppl):279–304 (discussion 304–305)
17. Blanke O et al (2000) Location of the human frontal eye field as defined by electrical cortical stimulation: anatomical, functional and electrophysiological characteristics. NeuroReport 11 (9):1907–1913
18. Fogassi L, Luppino G (2005) Motor functions of the parietal lobe. Curr Opin Neurobiol 15 (6):626–631
19. Blumenfeld H (2002) Neuroanatomy through clinical cases, vol xxii. Sinauer, Sunderland, p 951
20. Cushing H (1909) A note upon the faradic stimulation of the postcentral gyrus in conscious patients. Brain 32:10
21. Broca P (1865) On the seat of the faculty of articulate language. Bulletin Soc Anat Paris 6:57
22. Nolte J, Sundsten JW (2002) The human brain: an introduction to its functional anatomy, vol xiii, 5th edn. Mosby, St. Louis, p 650
23. Wernicke C (1874) Der aphasische Symptomencomplex. Kohn und Weigert, Breslau

24. Gatignol P et al (2004) Double dissociation between picture naming and comprehension: an electrostimulation study. NeuroReport 15(1):191–195
25. Nolte J (2009) The human brain: an introduction to its functional anatomy, vol xii, 6th edn. Mosby/Elsevier, Philadelphia, p 720
26. Dronkers NF (1996) A new brain region for coordinating speech articulation. Nature 384 (6605):159–161
27. Scarone P et al (2009) Agraphia after awake surgery for brain tumor: new insights into the anatomo-functional network of writing. Surg Neurol 72(3):223–241
28. Lucas TH 2nd, McKhann GM 2nd, Ojemann GA (2004) Functional separation of languages in the bilingual brain: a comparison of electrical stimulation language mapping in 25 bilingual patients and 117 monolingual control patients. J Neurosurg 101(3):449–457
29. Moritz-Gasser S, Duffau H (2009) Evidence of a large-scale network underlying language switching: a brain stimulation study. J Neurosurg 111(4):729–732
30. de Schotten M Thiebaut et al (2005) Direct evidence for a parietal-frontal pathway subserving spatial awareness in humans. Science 309(5744):2226–2228
31. Wallner KE et al (1989) Patterns of failure following treatment for glioblastoma multiforme and anaplastic astrocytoma. Int J Radiat Oncol Biol Phys 16(6):1405–1409
32. Bello L et al (2010) Intraoperative use of diffusion tensor imaging fiber tractography and subcortical mapping for resection of gliomas: technical considerations. Neurosurg Focus 28 (2):E6
33. Pfurtscheller G (1992) Event-related synchronization (ERS): an electrophysiological correlate of cortical areas at rest. Electroencephalogr Clin Neurophysiol 83(1):62–69
34. Eulitz C et al (1996) Oscillatory neuromagnetic activity induced by language and non-language stimuli. Brain Res Cogn Brain Res 4(2):121–132
35. Martino J et al (2011) Resting functional connectivity in patients with brain tumors in eloquent areas. Ann Neurol 69(3):521–532
36. Picht T et al (2011) Preoperative functional mapping for rolandic brain tumor surgery: comparison of navigated transcranial magnetic stimulation to direct cortical stimulation. Neurosurgery 69(3):581–588
37. Devlin JT, Watkins KE (2007) Stimulating language: insights from TMS. Brain 130(Pt 3): 610–622
38. Berger MS et al (1989) Brain mapping techniques to maximize resection, safety, and seizure control in children with brain tumors. Neurosurgery 25(5):786–792
39. Yingling CD et al (1999) Identification of motor pathways during tumor surgery facilitated by multichannel electromyographic recording. J Neurosurg 91(6):922–927
40. Duffau H, Denvil D, Capelle L (2002) Long term reshaping of language, sensory, and motor maps after glioma resection: a new parameter to integrate in the surgical strategy. J Neurol Neurosurg Psychiatry 72(4):511–516
41. Tate MC, Herbet G, Moritz-Gasser S, Tate JE, Duffau H (2014) Probabilistic map of critical functional regions of the human cerebral cortex: Broca's area revisited. Brain 137 (10):2773–2782
42. De Benedictis A, Sarubbo S, Duffau H (2012) Subcortical surgical anatomy of the lateral frontal region: human white matter dissection and correlations with functional insights provided by intraoperative direct brain stimulation: laboratory investigation. J Neurosurg 117 (6):1053–1069

Radiation Therapy of Glioblastoma

Igor J. Barani and David A. Larson

Abstract Glioblastoma multiforme (GBM) is the most common malignant brain tumor that affects approximately 17,000 patients annually. Clear survival advantages have been demonstrated with postoperative radiation therapy (RT) to doses of 5,000–6,000 cGy but dose-escalation attempts beyond 6,000 cGy have resulted in increased toxicity but no additional survival benefit. To improve local control and limit toxicity to normal brain tissue with these infiltrating tumors, novel imaging techniques are actively being explored to better define tumor extent and associated RT treatment fields. Hyperfractionated RT has been associated with a survival detriment. Current standard-of-care treatment involves concurrent use of temozolomide and RT to 6,000 cGy over 30 days followed by adjuvant temozolomide treatment for 6 months. Brachytherapy and stereotactic radiosurgery are effective therapies for relapsed GBM but tend to be associated with notable toxicity. More recently, re-irradiation strategies employ concurrent use of bevacizumab to limit treatment-related injury while still permitting delivery of meaningful doses. These clinical trials are ongoing and merits of these strategies are not yet clear but appear promising.

Keywords Radiation therapy · Glioblastoma · Radiation trials

Contents

I.J. Barani (✉) · D.A. Larson
Departments of Radiation Oncology and Neurological Surgery, University of California, 505 Parnassus Avenue, Room L08B, San Francisco, CA 94143–0226, USA
e-mail: baranii@radonc.ucsf.edu

D.A. Larson
e-mail: dlarson@radonc.ucsf.edu

J. Raizer and A. Parsa (eds.), *Current Understanding and Treatment of Gliomas*,
Cancer Treatment and Research 163, DOI 10.1007/978-3-319-12048-5_4

1 Introduction

Approximately half the 17,000 cases of central nervous system neoplasms diagnosed annually in the United States are categorized as glioblastoma multiforme (GBM). GBM represents the most aggressive subgroup of malignant gliomas, with a median survival of 6 months following surgical resection alone, and about 14–17 months in patients who undergo the most aggressive combined modality treatments [1, 2].

Radiation therapy (RT) has long been the standard adjuvant approach for glioblastoma, and it remains the primary treatment modality in unresectable glioblastoma. There is clear evidence for randomized trials supporting the benefit of post-resection RT [3–6], and other nominal forms of RT delivery. This chapter focuses on the evolution of RT in the treatment of glioblastoma, with the goal of providing a better understanding of the advances made and how these serve as foundation for future studies.

2 Establishing the Role of Post-resection RT

Early nonrandomized studies. The need for postoperative RT has been recognized given the infiltrative nature of glioblastoma, which makes complete surgical resection difficult without an unacceptable surgical neurologic morbidity. Early experience with postoperative RT was limited primarily to single-institution case series, many of which, prior to the 1960s, reported unimpressive and highly variable results. In many of these series, subtherapeutic doses of RT have been used (≤2000 cGy) [7–10]. The first large case series suggesting a survival advantage was reported by the Montréal Neurology Institute, in which patients received an average total dose of 5,000–6,000 cGy [11]. This was also the first report to include a central pathology review, which likely reduced the inclusion of anaplastic astrocytoma or other lower grade gliomas in the study.

There were other case series reported in the 1960s and 1970s that suggested a survival advantage with postoperative RT [7–13]. The interpretation of these early outcomes is complicated by the nonrandomized nature of these studies and inconsistencies in classification of glioblastoma. There were also significant variations in doses of RT, but in aggregate, survival trends with postoperative RT were favorable.

Early randomized studies. The Brain Tumor Study Group (BTSG; later renamed the Brain Tumor Cooperative Group (BTCG)) initiated several randomized studies

Table 1 Randomized studies of post-resection radiotherapy in glioblastoma

Trial	Patients (% GBM)	Treatment	Med. survival (months)	*P* value
BTSG 66-01 [4]	96 (85 %)	No radiotherapy	3.5	<0.05
		WBRT < 5000 cGy	7.7	
		WBRT ≥ 5000 cGy	8.4	
BTSG 69-01 [3]	222 (90 %)	No radiotherapy (BSC)	3.1	0.001
		WBRT 5000-6000 cGy	8.4	
		WBRT + BCNU	8.0	
		BCNU (no radiotherapy)	4.3	
BTSG 72-01 [6, 14]	358 (84 %)	CCNU (no radiotherapy)	7.2	NR
		WBRT 6000 cGY	8.4	
		WBRT + BCNU	11.9	
		WBRT + methyl-CCNU	7.2	

BCNU carmustine, *BSC* best supportive care, *GBM* glioblastoma multiforme, *NR* not reported, *WBRT* whole-brain radiotherapy

beginning in the 1970s that established postoperative RT as the standard of care in the treatment of GBM (Table 1). The first of the initial three studies (BTSG 66–01) randomized patients with newly diagnosed malignant gliomas after resection to mithramycin or no chemotherapy, with whole-brain radiotherapy (WBRT) being allowed. In all, 55 % of patients received WBRT, with approximately half receiving at least 3,000 cGy. This study showed no significant difference in median survival between patients treated with mithramycin or no chemotherapy, but those patients who received adjuvant WBRT were found to have a statistically significant survival advantage (8.4 vs. 3.5 months; $p < 0.05$). When outcomes were evaluated as a function of WBRT dose (either ≤5,000 cGy or >5,000 cGy), there was a strong trend toward improved survival favoring patients treated to a higher dose of WBRT. Interestingly, even patients treated to lower doses of WBRT had improved survival compared with those not receiving WBRT at all [4]. These data strongly suggested that inclusion of RT offers clinical benefit to patients with GBM.

The results of the BTSG 66–01 study led to a subsequent study in which RT was a randomized form of treatment. BTSG 69–01 randomized patients after surgical resection to receive the best supportive care (BSC) or chemotherapy (carmustine/BCNU) with or without WBRT. All therapeutic modalities demonstrated superiorly when compared to BSC with overall survival as a primary outcome. The BTSG investigators also noted that a significant cohort of patients treated with WBRT plus BCNU survived to 18 months, compared with the group receiving RT alone ($P = 0.01$) [3].

A follow-up study on BTSG 69–01 attempted to further evaluate the role of nitrosoureas plus RT (BTSG 72–01) [6, 14]. Patients received postoperative WBRT with or without a nitrosourea (BCNU or methyl-CCNU); those patients who received BCNU plus WBRT had the longest median survival. BTSG 72–01 prospectively confirmed the survival advantage observed in BTSG 69–01.

Additionally, both studies (BTSG 69–01 and 72–01) showed a trend toward improved survival. Again, there was a significant portion of patients who lived up to 18 months in a group that received chemotherapy (BCNU) plus RT. Although the benefit of postoperative RT was clearly established by these two studies, the benefit of adjuvant chemotherapy remained a question.

3 Determining Optimal RT Dose and Fractionation

Optimal radiation doses. A subsequent publication by BTCG retrospectively evaluated combined results from BTSG 66–01, 69–01, and 72–01, with special focus on whether dose escalation of RT improved survival [15]. Altogether, 621 evaluable patients were identified, of which 86 % were pathologically confirmed GBM cases, and the survival data was analyzed by subgroups based on the dose of WBRT received. Median survival times of only 4.2 and 3.1 months were reported for patients treated with less than 4,500 cGy or those who received no RT, respectively. Median survival durations of 6.5, 8.4, and 9.8 months were reported for patients treated with 5,000, 5,500, and 6,000 cGy, respectively. There was progressive improvement in survival with doses in excess of 5,000 cGy, with no statistically significant differences in toxicity observed between the 5,000 and 6,000 cGy treatment groups [15].

This apparent association between improved survival and RT doses ≥5,000 cGy shifted the clinical trial focus to further dose escalation of RT. Salazar and colleagues evaluated doses ranging from 6,000 to 8,000 cGy in three dose levels of WBRT, with and without local boost [16]. More than half the patients randomized to the highest dose level received a cumulative RT dose of 7,500 cGy or more. The study also included a retrospective cohort with then-conventional doses of WBRT (5,000–5,500 cGy). The actuarial median survival in the highest dose cohort (≥7,500 cGy) was 13 months compared to 9.8 months in the next highest dose group and only 7 months in the retrospective cohort treated with then-conventional WBRT. The survival difference between the highest dose cohort and then-conventional WBRT group reached statistical significance ($p < 0.05$). This statistical result should be interpreted with caution since prospective and retrospective patient outcomes were compared. Survival outcomes between prospectively treated patients at progressively escalated RT doses were not statistically significant, and survival curves for all dose groups were superimposable by 2 years [16].

Within this same study, autopsy data were reported for about 40 % of participating patients, including 10 autopsies from the highest dose cohort [16]. Autopsy specimens demonstrate regions of viable tumor within irradiated regions, even at the highest RT doses of 7,000–8,000 cGy. Additionally, marked radiation effect (e.g., necrosis) was seen microscopically in normal brain tissues at the periphery of the tumor. (*Note*: The authors did not comment on necrosis in other regions of the brain after WBRT.) These autopsy results, particularly the strong evidence of radiation necrosis at doses exceeding 6,000 cGy, suggested that dose escalation

Table 2 Median survival in RTOG 74-01/ECOG 1374 [17]

		Med. survival (months)	
Treatment	Patients	Overall	GBM subgroup
WBRT 6,000 cGy	141	9.3	8.7
WBRT 6,000 cGy + boost 1000 cGy	103	8.2	7.7
WBRT 6,000 cGy + BCNU	156	9.7	7.8
WBRT 6,000 cGy + methyl-CCNU + dacarbazine	138	10.1	9.2

BCNU carmustine, *GBM* glioblastoma multiforme, *WBRT* whole-brain radiotherapy

beyond this dose should be undertaken with caution. It is also worth noting that all of these studies were done in the pre-computer tomography (CT) and magnetic resonance imaging (MRI) era and toxicity assessments were largely based on clinical symptomatology and post-treatment autopsy results if available.

In an effort to further define the optimal dosing for post-resection RT (with or without chemotherapy), Chang and colleagues reported results from an intergroup trial evaluating standard WBRT to 6,000 cGy compared with escalated doses of RT [17, 18]. This phase III trial included four treatment arms: (1) WBRT (6,000 cGy), (2) WBRT + boost (6,000 cGy + 1,000 cGy), (3) WBRT (6,000 cGY) + BCNU, and (4) WBRT (6,000 cGy) + methyl-CCNU and dacarbazine (*Note*: Temozolamide is a prodrug and an imidazotetrazine derivative of the alkylating agent dacarbazine). Unlike the study conducted by Salazar and colleagues that included a retrospective WBRT cohort, the intergroup trial prospectively randomized patients to received then-standard doses of WBRT. In summary, the intergroup trial essentially demonstrated that escalation of RT doses above 6,000 cGy, or the addition of chemotherapy, did not significantly improve survival outcomes beyond WBRT alone to 6,000 cGy (Table 2), and subset analysis of patients with pathologically proved GBM revealed nonsignificant survival differences between the treatment groups ($p = 0.59$) [18]. Consistent with what has been previously reported in BTSG 69–01 and 72–01, the addition of current BCNU did not significantly improve overall or median survival, with the exception of a trend toward improved survival among the subgroup of patients less than 60 years of age, and a trend toward improved survival at 18 months. In this study, the 18-month survival rate among patients 40–60-years old was 10.3 % for 6,000 cGy WBRT versus 30.9 % for 6,000 cGy WBRT plus BCNU [18].

4 Determining the Optimal RT Field Size

Whole-brain versus involved-field RT. In the early treatments and clinical trials of glioblastoma, WBRT was utilized for treatment primarily because of concerns that glioblastoma may be a multicentric disease in a significant number of cases and that available radiologic techniques were inadequate in determining the extent and location of disease [19–22]. This assumption was subsequently challenged and it was shown that multicentric involvement with GBM is relatively uncommon. For example, Hochberg and Pruitt reported results of serial CT scans and correlative autopsy data in 35 GBM patients [22]. In their report, GBM was found to relapse within a 2 cm margin of the primary site in 90 % of cases, and only 6 % of patients treated with radiotherapy were found to have a multicentric disease at autopsy. Additionally, multiple subsequent studies have demonstrated that there is an upper limit to the WBRT dose in terms of both necrosis and cognitive dysfunction thresholds [23, 24]. Given this toxicity data and its association with high/escalated doses of WBRT is the observed local failure intensification of RT to a local tumor and a surrounding margin.

Beginning in the early 1970s, interest was generated in comparing outcomes of WBRT with involved-field RT (IFRT), where IFRT was defined as radiotherapy administered to the tumor and surrounding tissue encompassed by a 3 cm geometric margin around the tumor [25–28]. In a retrospective review of 127 patients who received RT for treatment of GBM, Onoyama and colleagues reported nearly identical 1-year survival rates with IFRT compared with WBRT [28]. Ramsey and Brand compared two prospectively randomized groups of GBM patients treated with WBRT (median dose = 4,400 cGy) or IFRT (median dose = 5,300 cGy), noting improved survival outcomes in patients treated with higher doses delivered to limited field [27]. In BTCG 80–01, patients with GBM were randomized to receive WBRT to a dose of 6,020 cGy or WBRT to 4300 cGy followed by IFRT boost to additional 1,720 cGy [24]. Survival differences between the treatment groups were not significantly different. Based on these data suggesting comparable outcomes with WBRT and IFRT, IFRT has become the standard of care in the treatment of GBM. This standard persists to this day.

Role of imaging in RT field design. Delivery of RT in the treatment of GBM cases is largely limited by difficulties in target definition/delineation. Although CT and MR imaging have improved the ability to deliver IFRT, these imaging modalities cannot reliably indicate regions of active, non-enhancing, or microscopic tumor. Furthermore, the conventional method used to identify tumor—assessments of gadolinium enhancement on MRI—is also a poor indicator of tumor (or recurrence in the posttreatment setting) after anti-VEGF (vascular endothelial growth factor) therapy, which is increasingly being used to treat patients with glioma. Several promising and novel imaging techniques are being investigated to provide better tumor definition. These will be briefly reviewed below even though their application in treatment planning and posttreatment evaluation varies considerably.

Magnetic resonance spectroscopy imaging (MRSI) is one such technique. MRSI provides information about tumor activity based on the levels of cellular metabolites such as choline, creatine, N-acetylaspartate, lactate, and lipid [29]. MRSI relies on the detection of alterations in these metabolite levels in predicting areas of occult disease; theoretically, targeting of these areas of an occult disease may decrease the rates of local recurrence [30, 31]. In one such early study, Graves and colleagues performed a retrospective study in which the prognostic value of MRSI was explored in patients with high-grade glioma treated with Gamma Knife radiation [31]. Patients without MRSI activity outside the areas of MRI contrast enhancement had significantly better outcomes than patients with MRSI activity outside the region of MRI contrast enhancement. In a follow-up study of 34 patients with high-grade gliomas, Pirzkall and colleagues found metabolically active tumors outside the region of enhancement (≤28 mm) on T2-weighted MRIs in 88 % of patients. Interestingly, MRIs in general predicted a larger volume of microscopic disease by 50 % or more compared with MRSI (using abnormality index of 2, 3, and 4), suggesting that targeted RT based on results of anatomic versus metabolic imaging would likely be of significantly different volumes and locations [30].

Another imaging modality under active investigation is diffusion-weighted MR imaging (DWI). In DWI, each voxel of the image has an intensity that reflects the rate of Brownian motion of water molecules or their diffusion rate in tissue at that location. The intensity of each voxel is quantified by calculating the apparent diffusion coefficient (ADC); that is, the right of water movement in mm^2/s. Different tissue types have different ADCs, and increased cellularity correlates with reduced ADC values. Areas of glioma/tumor are hypothesized to have lower ADC values than areas of normal brain, or radiation-induced treatment effects in the post-RT setting. The median ADC values for grade 3 and grade 4 gliomas are approximately 1.5 times that of normal appearing white matter within T2 lesion, with a trend toward lower values within contrast-enhancing lesions [32]. An analysis of the prognosis for 56 patients with untreated glioblastoma showed that both the presurgical values of the 10th percentile of ADC in contrast-enhancing lesions and the volume of the overall T2 lesions that exhibited ADC values less than 1.5 times that of normal appearing white matter were predictive of shorter overall survival [32]. These results are consistent with other published data and with the notion that the presence of regions with ADC values in the range of 1.0–1.5 times that of normal appearing white matter in contrast-enhancing lesions of glioblastoma are associated with a more cellular and aggressive phenotype [33–36]. Immediately after surgery, there are often regions of very low ADC close to the cavity that subsequently become enhancing and then disappear on follow-up examinations. In a recent analysis of 32 patients with GBM who had presurgical, immediate postsurgical, and pre-RT MR examinations, it was found that 21 of 32 patients showed reduced diffusion and 8 subsequently exhibited increased enhancement within a similar region that could have been confused with tumor progression [36]. This implies that the inclusion of diffusion-weighted imaging in the immediate postsurgical scan may be helpful in distinguishing between real and pseudo-progression, and may also be helpful in RT planning. It is also interesting to note that, when the pre-RT examination was taken as a new baseline scan for an expanded cohort patients with GBM, both the volume of the T2 lesion and the volume within the T2 lesion that showed ADC less than 1.5 times that of normal appearing white matter are predictors of poor overall survival, but the volume of the contrast enhancing lesion was not.

Diffusion tensor imaging (DTI) is a more complex version of DWI that can determine the directionality and magnitude of water diffusion, which is termed fractional anisotropy. Values for this parameter lie in the range of 0–1, and are high in normal white matter. DTI quantitates disorganization (damage) of white matter tracts, which is more likely in the lesions or radiation necrosis (or tumor necrosis) than in tumor recurrence because necrosis generally destroys these tracts, while tumor tends to displace or compress them. A case report of three patients found fractional anisotropy values of 0.27–0.29 for recurrent tumor and 0.17 for radiation necrosis, which suggested DTI might be able to distinguish recurrent tumor from necrosis [37]. A larger series will be needed to determine the utility of DTI in diagnosis of pre- and post-radiation enhancing lesions in patients with glioma. Currently, the utility of DTI in radiation treatment planning is unclear.

A number of MRI techniques have been applied to assess changes in microvasculature and to link variations in the estimated parameters with response to therapy. Their role in RT planning is less clear. The two methods most commonly used in the brain are dynamic contrast-enhanced (DCE) and dynamic susceptibility-weighted contrast (DSC) imaging. Several recent reviews have provided a thorough description of the methodology and examples patient data [29]. Briefly, DCE imaging takes advantage of the changes in the T1 associated with the passage of gadolinium through the vasculature and leakage into the extracellular space for regions in which the blood–brain barrier has been compromised [38–42]. When applying certain sampling techniques in conjunction with the latest parallel reconstructions strategies, time resolution of 5–10 s can be achieved for three-dimensional imaging sequence that covers an axial slab of 6–8 cm, partial brain volume. A number of different approaches have been applied to analyze the changes in signal intensity from these dynamic data and to estimate parameters such as the fractional blood volume *(f_BV) and permeability (K_ps* or K_trans_). The most widely used model is from Tofts and Kermode but other models are also in use today [38].

DSC imaging uses echoplanar sequences with a rapid bolus of gadolinium to assess changes in relaxivity within the vasculature and interstitial space with a 1–2 s time resolution [43]. The change in relaxivity is estimated as being proportional to the concentration of gadolinium. Within a particular region of interest, a decrease in the observed signal intensity usually corresponds to the arrival of the agent in the local vasculature. The changes in intensity are typically characterized by the peak height (PH), area under the curve relative to normal-appearing white matter (rCBV), and the percentage recovery (%REC) or recirculation factor (RF) [44].

Parametric maps that are derived from DCE and DSC imaging data have been proposed as noninvasive methods for predicting a tumor grade and assessing the response to therapy [45–48]. Although the presence of abnormal vasculature is known to be a histologically characteristic marker for glioblastoma, the magnitude and spatial extent of elevated rCBV in the initial presurgery scan were found to be predictive of overall survival [49]. One explanation for this is that, because the surgical resection is focused on the enhancing volume, it typically removes the majority of the region with increased vasculature. For patients with a residual vascular abnormality, conventional treatment with RT and temozolomide exhibits a short-term effect on the lesion, with a reduction in rCBV of a temporary increase in permeability. The magnitudes of these changes are reflected in the size of the contrast-enhancing lesion, with a lesion on the post-RT scan representing a balance between the two effects. In a recent study that followed a cohort of patients with glioblastoma through their initial treatment, it was found that although there was an association between progression-free survival and rCBV at pre-RT and post-RT examinations, none of the vascular parameters were related to overall survival [50]. Modern data that examine the effect of treatment, metabolic or other tumor parameters may be helpful in understanding the relationship between short-term changes in vasculature and long-term effects on the lesion as a whole. The ability to monitor changes in permeability and vascular density is expected to be critically important for the assessment of the impact of anti-angiogenic agents. In such cases, there is an ongoing debate about the most appropriate time points to detect the effect on MR parameters, and whether DCE or DSC techniques should be used to evaluate such changes.

Functional scanning, which uses PET to detect the breakdown of intravenously injected labeled compounds, has shown potential utility for identifying tumor recurrence. However, *18_F-fluorodeoxyglucose (FDG)-PET has limited sensitivity and specificity in distinguishing tumor from necrosis owing to the baseline high glucose utilization of the normal brain. Use of amino acid tracers derived from tyrosine and methionine overcomes the high background signal seen with a glucose-based PET, and can discriminate between tumor necrosis* [51]. *Furthermore, amino acid transport is energy-dependent and as such requires viable cells. The values of 75 % sensitivity and 75 % specificity were reported for* 11_C-methionine PET in a series of 26 patients [52]. Although these novel imaging techniques are of ongoing interest, they are yet to become a standard diagnostic approach in the evaluation and treatment planning of glioblastoma.

5 Dose Intensification: Brachytherapy, Radiosurgery, and Hyperfractionation

In an effort to improve outcomes and glioblastoma, various strategies were employed to locally intensify RT [53–55]. Such strategies have included less traditional forms of RT (brachytherapy, radiolabeled antibodies, radiosurgery), alternative dosing schedules (accelerated and hyperfractionated RT), and the use of radiosensitizing agents. Most of the dose intensification strategies (with the exception of radiosensitizer trials) will be reviewed below.

Brachytherapy. Interstitial delivery of RT, brachytherapy, directs radiation to well-defined tumor target, or resection bed, thereby sparing normal brain tissue from toxicity of high-dose RT and theoretically enabling local, high-dose treatment. Ample research has evaluated different means of delivering interstitial brachytherapy, leading to a debate as to whether radioisotopes should be implanted temporarily or permanently, and which radioisotopes are the most suitable for treatment of gliomas.

Some of the earliest brachytherapy reports from the 1980s focused on the treatment of locally relapsed glioma in patients who had previously received definitive RT [53, 54, 56–58]. Later, focus shifted to using brachytherapy as a local boost in conjunction with IFRT in cases of newly diagnosed glioblastoma [59–63].

A Northern California Oncology Group study (NCOG 6G–82–2) reported a remarkable median survival of 20.5 months in newly diagnosed GBM patients treated with *125_Iodine* (125_I) implants following 6,000 cGy of IFRT [59]. The study was criticized for not including a prospectively randomized comparison group of patients who received IFRT alone, and that patients with smaller, more peripherally located tumors were enrolled (e.g., selection bias). Additionally, 38 of the original 67 patients had been ineligible for the brachytherapy boost treatment after demonstrating no response or poor response to the initial IFRT. Consequently, the NCOG study reported on survival outcomes of the highly selected and most favorable patients enrolled in the study.

In contrast, Laperriere and colleagues in a Canadian study failed to demonstrate a significant survival advantage with 125_I implants following standard IFRT to 5,000 cGy [60]. It is difficult to interpret the outcomes of this study since the dose of IFRT was suboptimal. BTCG 87–01 evaluated survival in newly diagnosed malignant glioma patients (grade III and IV) patients treated with combination of BCNU and either IFRT or brachytherapy [64]. Median survival was not significantly different between the treatment groups, and no survival advantage was observed on subgroup analysis of patients with glioblastoma (Table 3).

In aggregate, the favorable survival results reported in single-arm (often single-institution) studies using brachytherapy as part of initial therapy for glioblastoma were not confirmed by randomized studies comparing brachytherapy with IFRT as part of the initial treatment regiment. It is worth noting that brachytherapy is not without complications and any perceived limited benefit needs to be weighed against the risk of potential complications of an invasive procedure. For example, Laperriere and colleagues reported 15 brachytherapy-related complications (out of 63 total patients) in their series, including neurologic decline requiring high-dose steroid treatment, intracerebral hemorrhage, exacerbation of seizures, infection, and arterial occlusion) [60]. Given the lack of prospective randomized study data to support the use of brachytherapy in the initial treatment of glioblastoma, its role in clinical practice (outside of the clinical trial setting) is primarily limited to the treatment of recurrent disease.

Table 3 Brachytherapy in newly diagnosed glioblastoma

Trial	Patients	Treatment	Med. survival (months)
NCOG 6G-82-2 [59]	29[a]	IFRT 6,000 cGy + ^{125}I implants	20.5
Laperriere et al. [60]	63	IFRT 5,000 cGy	13.2
		IFRT 5,000 cGy + ^{125}I implants	13.8
BTCG 87-01 [64]	270	IFRT 6,000 cGy + BCNU	13.7
		IFRT 6,000 cGy + ^{125}I implants + BCNU	15.8

BCNU = carmustine, IFRT = involved-field radiotherapy

[a] Survival outcomes reported for 29 of the original 67 patient cohort, 38 patients were excluded after failing to respond to initial IFRT

GliaSite. The GliaSite RT system (*Cytyc*) received FDA approval in 2001 as a novel method of brachytherapy delivery for the treatment of high-grade gliomas. The GliaSite is an expandable balloon catheter that is temporarily filled with radioactive *125*-I liquid through a subcutaneous reservoir after being placed into the resection cavity after tumor debulking. The balloon applicator conforms to the shape of the resection cavity and theoretically enables homogeneous dose delivery to the surrounding brain tissue. Since the applicator is placed at the time of surgery, there is no need for an additional surgical procedure to perform brachytherapy and, consequently, infection and perioperative risks are theoretically lower than would be expected for more traditional form of brain brachytherapy.

The New Approaches to Brain Tumor Therapy (NABTT) group conducted a trial of GliaSite in the treatment of recurrent malignant gliomas. Patients in the study received 4,000–6,000 cGy of dose to the resection cavity margin (target volume) via the GliaSite system. The observed median survival of 12.7 months was observed in this recurrent setting. These encouraging early results prompted further investigations of the GliaSite system in the upfront or newly diagnosed setting. Most of these more recent trials report survival outcomes that are comparable to historical data of other multi-modality treatments. There are no prospective, randomized studies of GliaSite in the treatment of malignant glioma [65, 66].

Radio-immunotherapy. This unique form of RT delivery involves the use of radiolabeled antibodies targeting malignant brain tissue. Investigators at Duke University have been studying the efficacy of a *131*-I-labeled murine anti-tenascin monoclonal antibody (*131*-I-m81C6) in the treatment of newly diagnosed and recurrent malignant brain tumors [67–79]. Tenascin is an extracellular matrix glycoprotein expressed ubiquitously in multiple tumor types, including high-grade gliomas, but not in normal brain tissue. The murine monoclonal immunoglobulin G2b (81C6) binds to an epitope within tenascin, resulting in inhibition and delay of cell growth. Administration of radiolabeled antibody (*131*-I-m81C6) involves direct injection of the antibody into the resection cavity at the time of tumor resection.

A phase II study of newly diagnosed glioma patients treated with *131*-I-m81C6 followed by conventional IFRT and chemotherapy reported a median survival of 20 months, with a median survival of 18 months in patients with GBM [71]. A more recent study of *131*-I-m81C6 in cases of recurrent malignant brain tumors reported a median survival of 15 months in a subgroup of patients with GBM and gliosarcoma [74]. This phase II experience yielded survival results comparable to or more favorable than what has been reported with other salvage therapies, including temozolamide, stereotactic radiosurgery, interstitial chemotherapy, and brachytherapy. In addition, the rates of radiation necrosis in the phase II trials of *131*-I-m81C6 were lower than those observed with other dose intensification methods [67]. However, these survival results and rates of neurotoxicity must be interpreted in the context of the overall good performance status of the patient groups analyzed; most patients (>90 %) had Karnofsky performance status (KSP) scores >80. Variations in neurotoxicity can be explained by marked variance in the radiation doses delivered to the 2-cm surgical cavity resection margin [73]. A phase III study is being planned at Duke to follow-up on these encouraging results using patient-specific dosimetry as well as antibody dosing.

Stereotactic Radiosurgery (SRS). Stereotactic radiosurgery involves the precise delivery of high radiation dose in 1–5 treatments. Both frame-based and frameless stereotactic systems were used in the treatment of malignant glioma, with the earliest application being in 1968. Skepticism over the technology and cost constraints resulted in generally slow acceptance by the mainstream oncology community. Traditionally, radiosurgery was delivered with a Gamma Knife device using multiple non-coplanar isocentric *60*-Cobalt sources, but more recently, linear accelerator (linac)-based approaches are also becoming popular due to their greater versatility. With the advances in both hardware and software, radiosurgery became increasingly used to treat brain metastases in the 1980s and, shortly thereafter, has also been applied to recurrent glioma treatments.

SRS involves the use of numerous beamlets of radiation aimed precisely at an immobilized target to deliver high-dose, usually ablative dose, of radiation. Although no single beamlet carries significant energy, a large dose is deposited at the intersection of these beamlets, with a steep dose falloff outside the target. As tumor size increases, this falloff becomes shallower and contact surface with the surrounding tissue greater, and typically radiosurgery becomes prohibitive with tumors in excess of 4–5 cm diameter using a single-session treatment. For larger lesions, most practitioners opt to split the treatment up over 3 or 5 fractions, delivering moderate doses at each session. This approach theoretically preserves the biological effectiveness of the treatment while minimizing normal tissue effects in the surrounding brain that would otherwise be unacceptable with single-session treatment to a large target.

Several early retrospective reports of SRS in the setting of recurrent gliomas suggested a survival advantage with the addition of SRS. The suggestion of SRS use in malignant gliomas was first reported by Larson and colleagues from the University of California, San Francisco in 1990 [80]. Subsequently, Loeffler and colleagues from the Joint Center in Boston reported on a 37-patient series where radiosurgery was part of the initial treatment of malignant glioma [81]. After a median follow-up of 19 months, only 24 % of patients died of recurrent tumor (six, all with GBM), whereas two died of complications related to radiosurgery. All others eventually progressed outside of the radiosurgery field. A retrospective study from the University of Maryland comparing survival data in GBM patients treated with IFRT followed by SRS as a local boost treatment or SRS at the time of progression (salvage treatment) found that median survivals favored the group receiving SRS as a boost (25 vs. 13 months; $P = 0.0335$) [82]. RT Oncology Group (RTOG) study 93–05 evaluated SRS in a randomized study of 203 patients with GBM who received either conventional IFRT (6,000 cGy) plus BCNU or SRS prior to IFRT plus BCNU [83]. This study did not find any significant differences in median survival (13.5 months for SRS vs. 13.6 months for conventional IFRT), 2-year overall survival, quality-of-life deterioration, or cognitive decline [84]. Therefore, outside of the clinical trial setting, there is no clear indication for the use of SRS in the treatment of newly diagnosed GBM.

Fractionated stereotactic radiotherapy (FSRT). Stereotactic radiotherapy involves precisely targeted delivery of radiation using moderate doses over five or more treatments. RTOG 98–03 investigated escalated doses of FSRT in newly diagnosed GBM patients, with patients receiving IFRT to 4,600 cGy followed by FSRT boost to total doses of 6,600–8,400 cGy [85]. The acute- and late-toxicity date in this study were promising (no difference between grade 3 or 4 toxicities) at escalated dose levels of RT. Similar proportions of patients at each dose level required second resections.

Subsequently, the RTOG reported its phase II experience with administering accelerated RT with weekly stereotactic conformal boosts in 76 patients with newly diagnosed GBM (RTOG 00–23) [86]. During the course of standard RT to 5,000 cGy, patients received four weekly FSRT boosts (500 or 700 cGy per fraction), for a total cumulative dose of 7,000–7,800 cGy. Although reported toxicities were manageable, the median survival of 12.5 months was not improved compared with the RTOG historical database [86, 87]. However, a trend for improved survival was observed in subgroups of patients undergoing gross total resection (median survival of 16.1 vs. 12.0 months; $p = 0.19$). Additionally, a subgroup of patients classified as having more favorable disease according to a recursive partitioning analysis (RPA) model proposed by Curran and colleagues were noted to have improved median survival (14.7 months for RPA class IV patients vs. 11.3 months for the overall study cohort; $p = 0.15$) [86, 87].

Hyperfractionated and Accelerated Radiotherapy. Hyperfractionation involves more frequent (more than once daily; so-called conventional fractionation) administration of RT doses in an attempt to attain several theoretical radiobiologic advantages, including reduction in late radiation injury and prevention of tumor repopulation between treatments [88, 89]. Additionally, small and frequent doses of RT may redistribute dividing tumor cell population such that some tumor cells can be "forced" to enter more radiosensitive parts of the cell cycle. Thus, hyperfractioned RT (HFRT) offers the potential advantage of being able to give higher cumulative doses of RT without significant added toxicity [88, 89].

Much of the experience with HFRT in glioblastoma has not resulted in reports of survival advantage compared with standard or more conventionally fractionated RT. For example, the European Organization for the Research and Treatment of Cancer (EORTC) reported its experience with administering accelerated HFRT to doses of 4,200–6,000 cGy in 200 cGy-fractions given three times daily. An overall survival of 8.7 months was observed, with no differences in survival noted among any of the dose levels administered [90]. Several other groups reported similar results with accelerated HFRT failing to achieve significant improvements in median survival over conventional IFRT (Table 4).

In contrast with these data, RTOG 83–02 study results suggested a promising role for HFRT in the treatment of glioblastoma [91]. Patients were randomized to either HFRT or accelerated HFRT (AHFRT), with median survivals of 10.8 and 12.7 months reported (Table 4). However, survival outcomes in the subgroup of patients with GBM receiving higher HFRT doses of 7,680 and 8,160 cGy were superior to the survival outcomes observed in patients in the AHFRT group.

Table 4 Trials of hyperfractionated and accelerated radiotherapy in glioblastoma

Trial	Patients	Treatment	Med. survival (months)
EORTC [90]	66	200 cGy twice daily to:	8.7
		4,200 cGy	
		4,800 cGy	
		5,400 cGy	
		6,000 cGy	
Lutterbach et al. [109]	149	150 cGy thrice daily to:	8.8
		5,400 cGy	
Neider et al. [110]	126	130 cGy twice daily to:	7–10
		7,800 cGy	
		150 cGy twice daily to:	
		6,000 cGy	
Prados et al. [111]	231	AHFRT ± DFMO	8.6–9.8
		160 cGy twice daily to:	
		7040 cGy	
		Standard RT ± DFMO	
		180 cGy once daily to:	
		5,940 cGy	
RTOG 83-02 [91]	786	HFRT, 120 cGy twice daily to:	10.8–12.7[a]
		6,480 cGy	
		7,200 cGy	
		7,680 cGy	
		8,160 cGy	
		AHFRT, 160 cGy twice daily to:	
		4,800 cGy	
		5,440 cGy	
RTOG 90-06 [92, 93]	712	HFRT + BCNU	19.8[b]
		120 cGy twice daily to:	
		7,200 cGy	
		Standard RT + BCNU	21.9[b]
		200 cGy once daily to:	
		6,000 cGy	

AHFRT accelerated hyperfractionated radiation therapy, *BCNU* carmustine, *DFMO* difluoromethylornithine, *HFRT* hyperfractionated radiation therapy

[a] Subgroups with GBM treated with HFRT at higher doses of 7680 cGy and 8160 cGy had better survival than GBM patients treated with AFHRT

[b] Survival data reported in GBM subgroup ≤50-years old ($p = 0.05$)

RTOG 90–06 was initiated specifically to address whether higher doses of HFRT offered benefit over standard doses (6000 cGy) and fractionation with IFRT in glioblastoma. In this important phase III study, patients were randomized to

HFRT (120 cGy given twice daily to 7200 cGy) plus BCNU versus conventional IFRT (6000 cGy) plus BCNU [92, 93]. Ultimately, there was no survival advantage with HFRT, and in fact, the outcomes of patients treated with conventional IFRT to 6000 cGy were superior for patients 50 years of age or older (median survival of 21.9 and 19.8 months; $p = 0.05$); this trend was also observed on subgroup analysis of patients with GBM [92, 93].

6 Radiation Modulators/Sensitizers

Radiosensitizers or radiation modulators are usually systemic agents, typically chemotherapy or targeted agents that enhance the efficacy of RT. While comprehensive review of trials of radiation modulators is beyond the scope of this review, it is worth highlighting several trials that established current treatment standard.

As early RT trial experiences demonstrate (see above), the addition of chemotherapy, mainly nitrosoureas, did not statistically improve survival compared with patients receiving RT alone. At 2 years, fewer than 10 % of patients were alive [6]. Subsequent meta-analyses of randomized trials of radiation versus radiation plus nitrosourea-containing regimen showed only a modest improvement in 1-year survival outcomes in patients who received combination therapy [94, 95]. However, Stupp and colleagues performed a phase II trial in patients with newly diagnosed glioblastoma, administering daily lower dose temozolomide (75 mg/m2) during the course of RT, followed by 6 months of adjuvant, higher dose temozolomide at a single agent dose of 150–200 mg/m^2 for days 1–5 of a 28-day cycle [96]. The results of this phase II study were promising, demonstrating an overall median survival of 16 months.

These data led to a confirmatory, phase III study that was performed by the EORTC and the National Cancer Institute of Canada (NCIC) [97]. Newly diagnosed GBM patients were randomized to receive RT alone or concurrent RT + temozolomide followed by 6 months of adjuvant temozolomide. The study demonstrated a statistically significant improvement in median survival for the combined treatment arm (12.1 vs. 14.6 months) as well as a significant increase in 2-year survivors (10 % vs. 26 %) favoring the combined treatment cohort. Additionally, 88 % of patients completed the concurrent phase of treatment and 40 % received full 6 adjuvant cycles of chemotherapy. Tumor progression was still the most common reason for treatment cessation. The treatment was also well tolerated with an incidence of grade 3 or 4 hematologic toxicity of <4 % [97]. Because of these results, this chemoradiation regimen has been widely accepted as the new standard of care for patients with newly diagnosed GBM.

An update from this trial was presented at the 2007 meeting of the American Society of Radiation Oncology (ASTRO), demonstrating a 10 % 5-year survival rate in patients treated with the chemoradiation regimen and providing additional evidence of the efficacy of this therapy [98].

7 Re-irradiation for Recurrent Glioblastoma

There has been a long experience with re-irradiation of recurrent glioblastoma, however, recent observations that bevacizumab may have radioprotective effects rekindled interest in combined re-irradiation approaches. The combination of bevacizumab with re-irradiation increases the therapeutic ratio through increased antitumor and antivascular effects [99]. Preclinical data suggest that vascular endothelial growth factor (VEGF) is upregulated following radiation exposure, and therefore combination of anti-angiogenic agents with radiation may sensitize both tumors and associated tumor vasculature to RT [100]. Other preclinical models suggest that anti-angiogenic agents may specifically target the radioresistant and highly tumorigenic cancer stem cells by disrupting vascular niches harboring these fragile cancer stem cells [101]. Due to its vascular stabilization effects, bevacizumab may also be radioprotective and reduce the toxicity associated with re-irradiation by reducing the risk of radiation necrosis [102, 103].

Preliminary clinical evidence suggests improved outcome with the addition of concurrent and adjuvant bevacizumab to re-irradiation. Gutin and colleagues published results of 25 patients with recurrent grade III and IV gliomas using FSRT and concurrent bevacizumab; with a reported 6-month progression-free survival of 65 % and median overall survival of 12.5 months [104]. Median time to re-irradiation was 15 months. Enhancing tumor volume was ≤3.5 cm in maximum diameter. Treatments were well tolerated and there was no incidence of radiation necrosis and no additional need for corticosteroids following re-irradiation.

Similarly, a group from Duke University reported their institutional retrospective data on 63 patients with recurrent high-grade gliomas, including 49 glioblastoma patients treated with re-irradiation using SRS techniques combined with bevacizumab therapy [105]. The combined re-treatment was well tolerated and median time to re-irradiation was 19.6 months. Mean number of systemic therapies prior to SRS was 3.6 and mean number of therapies following SRS was 2.9. Median target volume was 4.8 cc. The 1-year overall survival in glioblastoma patients who received adjuvant (concurrent with or after SRS) bevacizumab was 50 % versus 22 % for patients not receiving adjuvant bevacizumab (p = 0.005). Both age <50 years and KPS >70 were associated with improved overall survival.

Niyazi and colleagues reported their single-institution experience in high-grade glioma patients treated with FSRT to 3,600 cGy in 18 daily fractions with concurrent bevacizumab, followed by maintenance bevacizumab [106]. Overall survival appeared to be improved in patients who received bevacizumab (12.1 months) compared to those who received either re-irradiation alone or re-irradiation with concurrent temozolomide (8.0 months). Treatment was well tolerated with no incidence of radiation necrosis and only one case of wound dehiscence. In aggregate, these preliminary results stimulated interest within RTOG to conduct a phase II trial of concurrent bevacizumab and re-irradiation versus bevacizumab alone as treatment for recurrent glioblastoma (RTOG 1205). This trial is currently open for enrollment.

We are conducting a similar dose-escalation study in the recurrent setting for patients with glioblastoma where FSRT techniques are used to re-irradiate target volumes up to 40 cc with concurrent bevacizumab therapy. Patients are currently being treated at a dose level of 3300 cGy (given over 3 fractions, every other day). Thus far, no grade 3 or higher treatment-related toxicities were observed during dose escalation that would preclude application of this technique and continued dose escalation. This study is ongoing.

8 Conclusion

Although the overall survival of patients with glioblastoma has not improved dramatically over the last several decades, there have been steady advances in utilization of combined modality treatments to improve survival rates while preserving acceptable quality of life among patients. Agents such as temozolomide have demonstrated modest survival advantage in combination with RT, but they helped us become more aware of aspects of the underlying tumor biology that lead to improved survival outcomes [107, 108]. These insights are already starting to lead to more appropriate therapeutic selection based on molecular profiles of individual patients.

Ongoing research with novel imaging techniques may allow for better targeting of occult tumor, and new techniques of delivering RT will continue to be explored as means of improving local dose intensification. With the advent of targeted therapies, rational combinations of chemotherapy and targeted agents for treatment of GBM are being developed based on unique tumor- and patient-molecular profiles. Rapid evaluation of these rational treatment approaches for efficacy will be aided by high-quality historical treatment outcomes data, such as the recursive partitioning analysis proposed by Curran and colleagues [87], against which new outcomes can be measured before being investigated in expensive phase III studies. These multiple avenues of research in glioblastoma show significant promise for future translation into substantial gains in patient outcomes.

References

1. Wilson TA, Karajannis MA, Harter DH (2014) Glioblastoma multiforme: state of the art and future therapeutics. Surg Neurol Int 5:64. doi:10.4103/2152-7806.132138
2. Omuro A, DeAngelis LM (2013) Glioblastoma and other malignant gliomas: a clinical review. JAMA 310(17):1842–1850. doi:10.1001/jama.2013.280319
3. Walker MD, Alexander E, Hunt WE, MacCarty CS, Mahaley MS, Mealey J, Norrell HA, Owens G, Ransohoff J, Wilson CB, Gehan EA, Strike TA (1978) Evaluation of BCNU and/or radiotherapy in the treatment of anaplastic gliomas. A cooperative clinical trial. J Neurosurg 49(3):333–343. doi:10.3171/jns.1978.49.3.0333

4. Walker MD, Alexander E, Hunt WE, Leventhal CM, Mahaley MS, Mealey J, Norrell HA, Owens G, Ransohoff J, Wilson CB, Gehan EA (1976) Evaluation of mithramycin in the treatment of anaplastic gliomas. J Neurosurg 44(6):655–667. doi:10.3171/jns.1976.44.6.0655
5. Walker MD, Hurwitz BS (1970) BCNU (1,3-bis(2-chloroethyl)-1-nitrosourea; NSC-409962) in the treatment of malignant brain tumor–a preliminary report. Cancer Chemother Rep 54 (4):263–271
6. Walker MD, Green SB, Byar DP, Alexander E Jr, Batzdorf U, Brooks WH, Hunt WE, MacCarty CS, Mahaley MS Jr, Mealey J Jr, Owens G, Ransohoff J 2nd, Robertson JT, Shapiro WR, Smith KR Jr, Wilson CB, Strike TA (1980) Randomized comparisons of radiotherapy and nitrosoureas for the treatment of malignant glioma after surgery. N Engl J Med 303(23):1323–1329. doi:10.1056/NEJM198012043032303
7. Sheline GE (1977) Radiation therapy of brain tumors. Cancer 39(2 Suppl):873–881
8. Schulz MD, Wang C-C, Zinninger GF, Tefft M (1968) Radiotherapy of intracranial neoplasms, with a special section on the radiotherapeutic management of central nervous system tumors in children. Prog Neurol Surg 2:318–370
9. Lindgren M (1953) Roentgen treatment of gliomata. Acta Radiol (Old series) 40 (2–3):325–334
10. Bouchard J, Peirce CB (1960) Radiation therapy in the management of neoplasms of the central nervous system, with a special note in regard to children-20 years experience, 1939–1958. Am J Roentgenol Radium Ther Nucl Med 84(4):610–628
11. Uihlein A, Colby MY, Layton DD, Parsons WR, Garter TL (1966) Comparison of surgery and surgery plus irradiation in the treatment of supratentorial gliomas. Acta Radiol 5 (1):67–78
12. Kramer S (1972) Proceedings: radiation therapy in the management of malignant gliomas. In: Proceedings of national cancer conference, vol 7. pp 823–826
13. Stage WS, Stein JJ (1974) Treatment of malignant astrocytomas. Am J Roentgenol 120 (1):7–18
14. Walker MD, Strike TA (1976) Evaluation of methyl CCNU, BCNU and Radiotherapy in Treatment of Malignant Glioma. In: Proceedings of the American Association for Cancer Research, vol MAR. pp 163–163
15. Walker MD, Strike TA, Sheline GE (1979) An analysis of dose-effect relationship in the radiotherapy of malignant gliomas. Int J Radiat Oncol Biol Phys 5(10):1725–1731
16. Salazar OM, Rubin P, Feldstein ML, Pizzutiello R (1979) High dose radiation therapy in the treatment of malignant gliomas: final report. Int J Radiat Oncol Biol Phys 5(10):1733–1740
17. Nelson DF, Diener-West M, Horton J, Chang CH, Schoenfeld D, Nelson JS (1988) Combined modality approach to treatment of malignant gliomas–re-evaluation of RTOG 7401/ECOG 1374 with long-term follow-up: a joint study of the radiation therapy oncology group and the eastern cooperative oncology group. NCI Monogr 6:279–284
18. Chang CH, Horton J, Schoenfeld D, Salazer O, Perez-Tamayo R, Kramer S, Weinstein A, Nelson JS, Tsukada Y (1983) Comparison of postoperative radiotherapy and combined postoperative radiotherapy and chemotherapy in the multidisciplinary management of malignant gliomas. A joint radiation therapy oncology group and eastern cooperative oncology group study. Cancer 52(6):997–1007
19. Salazar OM, Rubin P (1976) The spread of glioblastoma multiforme as a determining factor in the radiation treated volume. Int J Radiat Oncol Biol Phys 1(7–8):627–637
20. Concannon JP, Kramer S, Berry R (1960) The extent of intracranial gliomata at autopsy and its relationship to techniques used in radiation therapy of brain tumors. Am J Roentgenol Radium Ther Nucl Med 84:99–107
21. Salazar OM, Rubin P, McDonald JV, Feldstein ML (1976) Patterns of failure in intracranial astrocytomas after irradiation: analysis of dose and field factors. AJR Am J Roentgenol 126 (2):279–292. doi:10.2214/ajr.126.2.279
22. Hochberg FH, Pruitt A (1980) Assumptions in the radiotherapy of glioblastoma. Neurology 30(9):907–911. doi:10.1212/WNL.30.9.907

23. Marks JE, Baglan RJ, Prassad SC, Blank WF (1981) Cerebral radionecrosis: incidence and risk in relation to dose, time, fractionation and volume. Int J Radiat Oncol Biol Phys 7 (2):243–252
24. Shapiro WR, Green SB, Burger PC, Mahaley MS Jr, Selker RG, VanGilder JC, Robertson JT, Ransohoff J, Mealey J Jr, Strike TA et al (1989) Randomized trial of three chemotherapy regimens and two radiotherapy regimens and two radiotherapy regimens in postoperative treatment of malignant glioma. Brain tumor cooperative group trial 8001. J Neurosurg 71 (1):1–9. doi:10.3171/jns.1989.71.1.0001
25. Schryver AD, Greitz T, Forsby N, Brun A (1976) Localized shaped field radiotherapy of malignant glioblastoma multiforme. Int J Radiat Oncol Biol Phys 1(7–8):713–716
26. Caldwell WL, Aristizabal SA (1975) Treatment of glioblastoma multiforme: a review. Acta Radiol Ther Phys Biol 14(6):505–512
27. Ramsey RG, Brand WN (1973) Radiotherapy of glioblastoma multiforme. J Neurosurg 39 (2):197–202. doi:10.3171/jns.1973.39.2.0197
28. Onoyama Y, Abe M, Yabumoto E, Sakamoto T, Nishidai T (1976) Radiation therapy in the treatment of glioblastoma. AJR Am J Roentgenol 126(3):481–492. doi:10.2214/ajr.126.3.481
29. Nelson SJ (2011) Assessment of therapeutic response and treatment planning for brain tumors using metabolic and physiological MRI. NMR Biomed 24(6):734–749. doi:10.1002/nbm.1669
30. Pirzkall A, McKnight TR, Graves EE, Carol MP, Sneed PK, Wara WW, Nelson SJ, Verhey LJ, Larson DA (2001) Mr-spectroscopy Guided Target Delineation for High-grade Gliomas. Int J Radiat Oncol Biol Phys 50(4):915–928. doi:10.1016/S0360-3016(01)01548-6
31. Graves EE, Nelson SJ, Vigneron DB, Chin C, Verhey L, McDermott M, Larson D, Sneed PK, Chang S, Prados MD, Lamborn K, Dillon WP (2000) A preliminary study of the prognostic value of proton magnetic resonance spectroscopic imaging in gamma knife radiosurgery of recurrent malignant gliomas. Neurosurgery 46(2):319–326 (discussion 326–318). doi:10.1097/00006123-200002000-00011
32. Chang SM, Nelson S, Vandenberg S, Cha S, Prados M, Butowski N, McDermott M, Parsa AT, Aghi M, Clarke J, Berger M (2009) Integration of preoperative anatomic and metabolic physiologic imaging of newly diagnosed glioma. J Neurooncol 92(3):401–415. doi:10.1007/s11060-009-9845-0
33. Yamasaki F, Kurisu K, Satoh K, Arita K, Sugiyama K, Ohtaki M, Takaba J, Tominaga A, Hanaya R, Yoshioka H, Hama S, Ito Y, Kajiwara Y, Yahara K, Saito T, Thohar MA (2005) Apparent diffusion coefficient of human brain tumors at MR imaging. Radiology 235 (3):985–991. doi:10.1148/radiol.2353031338
34. Lam WW, Poon WS, Metreweli C (2002) Diffusion Mr imaging in glioma: does it have any role in the pre-operation determination of grading of glioma? Clin Radiol 57(3):219–225. doi:10.1053/crad.2001.0741
35. Teshima T, Inoue T, Ikeda H, Miyata Y, Nishiyama K, Murayama S, Yamasaki H, Kozuka T (1993) High-dose rate and low-dose rate intracavitary therapy for carcinoma of the uterine cervix. Final results of Osaka University Hospital. Cancer 72(8):2409–2414
36. Pirzkall A, McGue C, Saraswathy S, Cha S, Liu R, Vandenberg S, Lamborn KR, Berger MS, Chang SM, Nelson SJ (2009) Tumor regrowth between surgery and initiation of adjuvant therapy in patients with newly diagnosed glioblastoma. Neuro Oncol 11(6):842–852. doi:10.1215/15228517-2009-005
37. Kashimura H, Inoue T, Beppu T, Ogasawara K, Ogawa A (2007) Diffusion tensor imaging for differentiation of recurrent brain tumor and radiation necrosis after radiotherapy—three case reports. Clin Neurol Neurosurg 109(1):106–110. doi:10.1016/j.clineuro.2006.04.005
38. Tofts PS, Kermode AG (1991) Measurement of the blood-brain barrier permeability and leakage space using dynamic MR imaging. 1. Fundamental concepts. Magn Reson Med 17 (2):357–367

39. Harrer JU, Parker GJM, Haroon HA, Buckley DL, Embelton K, Roberts C, Balériaux D, Jackson A (2004) Comparative study of methods for determining vascular permeability and blood volume in human gliomas. J Magn Reson Imaging 20(5):748–757. doi:10.1002/jmri.20182
40. Ferl GZ, Xu L, Friesenhahn M, Bernstein LJ, Barboriak DP, Port RE (2010) An automated method for nonparametric kinetic analysis of clinical DCE-MRI data: application to glioblastoma treated with bevacizumab. Magn Reson Med 63(5):1366–1375. doi:10.1002/mrm.22335
41. Ashton E, Raunig D, Ng C, Kelcz F, McShane T, Evelhoch J (2008) Scan-rescan variability in perfusion assessment of tumors in MRI using both model and data-derived arterial input functions. J Magn Reson Imaging 28(3):791–796. doi:10.1002/jmri.21472
42. Evelhoch J, Garwood M, Vigneron D, Knopp M, Sullivan D, Menkens A, Clarke L, Liu G (2005) Expanding the use of magnetic resonance in the assessment of tumor response to therapy: workshop report, vol 65. Cancer Research, United States. doi:10.1158/0008-5472.CAN-05-0674
43. Rosen BR, Belliveau JW, Chien D (1989) Perfusion imaging by nuclear magnetic resonance. Magn Reson Q 5(4):263–281
44. Boxerman JL, Schmainda KM, Weisskoff RM (2006) Relative cerebral blood volume maps corrected for contrast agent extravasation significantly correlate with glioma tumor grade, whereas uncorrected maps do not. AJNR Am J Neuroradiol 27(4):859–867
45. Lupo JM, Banerjee S, Hammond KE, Kelley DAC, Xu D, Chang SM, Vigneron DB, Majumdar S, Nelson SJ (2009) GRAPPA-based susceptibility-weighted imaging of normal volunteers and patients with brain tumor at 7 T. Magn Reson Imaging 27(4):480–488. doi:10.1016/j.mri.2008.08.003
46. Barajas RF, Chang JS, Segal MR, Parsa AT, McDermott MW, Berger MS, Cha S (2009) Differentiation of recurrent glioblastoma multiforme from radiation necrosis after external beam radiation therapy with dynamic susceptibility-weighted contrast-enhanced perfusion MR imaging. Radiology 253(2):486–496. doi:10.1148/radiol.2532090007
47. Cha S, Tihan T, Crawford F, Fischbein NJ, Chang S, Bollen A, Nelson SJ, Prados M, Berger MS, Dillon WP (2005) Differentiation of low-grade oligodendrogliomas from low-grade astrocytomas by using quantitative blood-volume measurements derived from dynamic susceptibility contrast-enhanced MR imaging. AJNR Am J Neuroradiol 26(2):266–273
48. Law M, Yang S, Wang H, Babb JS, Johnson G, Cha S, Knopp EA, Zagzag D (2003) Glioma grading: sensitivity, specificity, and predictive values of perfusion MR imaging and proton MR spectroscopic imaging compared with conventional MR imaging. AJNR Am J Neuroradiol 24(10):1989–1998
49. Crawford FW, Khayal IS, McGue C, Saraswathy S, Pirzkall A, Cha S, Lamborn KR, Chang SM, Berger MS, Nelson SJ (2008) Relationship of Pre-surgery metabolic and physiological Mr imaging parameters to survival for patients with untreated GBM. J Neurooncol. doi:10.1007/s11060-008-9719-x
50. Li Y, Lupo JM, Polley M-Y, Crane JC, Bian W, Cha S, Chang S, Nelson SJ (2011) Serial analysis of imaging parameters in patients with newly diagnosed glioblastoma multiforme. Neuro Oncol 13(5):546–557. doi:10.1093/neuonc/noq194
51. Tsuyuguchi N, Takami T, Sunada I, Iwai Y, Yamanaka K, Tanaka K, Nishikawa M, Ohata K, Torii K, Morino M, Nishio A, Hara M (2004) Methionine positron emission tomography for differentiation of recurrent brain tumor and radiation necrosis after stereotactic radiosurgery—in malignant glioma. Ann Nucl Med 18(4):291–296
52. Terakawa Y, Tsuyuguchi N, Iwai Y, Yamanaka K, Higashiyama S, Takami T, Ohata K (2008) Diagnostic accuracy of 11C-methionine PET for differentiation of recurrent brain tumors from radiation necrosis after radiotherapy. J Nucl Med 49(5):694–699. doi:10.2967/jnumed.107.048082
53. Gutin PH, Phillips TL, Wara WM, Leibel SA, Hosobuchi Y, Levin VA, Weaver KA, Lamb S (1984) Brachytherapy of recurrent malignant brain tumors with removable high-activity iodine-125 sources. J Neurosurg 60(1):61–68. doi:10.3171/jns.1984.60.1.0061

54. Gutin PH, Leibel SA, Wara WM, Choucair A, Levin VA, Philips TL, Silver P, Da Silva V, Edwards MS, Davis RL (1987) Recurrent malignant gliomas: survival following interstitial brachytherapy with high-activity iodine-125 sources. J Neurosurg 67(6):864–873. doi:10.3171/jns.1987.67.6.0864
55. Selker RG, Shapiro WR, Burger P, Blackwood MS, Arena VC, Gilder JC, Malkin MG, Mealey JJ, Neal JH, Olson J, Robertson JT, Barnett GH, Bloomfield S, Albright R, Hochberg FH, Hiesiger E, Green S, Brain Tumor Cooperative Group (2002) The Brain Tumor Cooperative Group NIH Trial 87-01: a randomized comparison of surgery, external radiotherapy, and carmustine versus surgery, interstitial radiotherapy boost, external radiation therapy, and carmustine. Neurosurgery 51(2):343–355 (discussion 355–347)
56. Hosobuchi Y, Phillips TL, Stupar TA, Gutin PH (1980) Interstitial brachytherapy of primary brain tumors: preliminary report. J Neurosurg 53(5):613–617. doi:10.3171/jns.1980.53.5.0613
57. Gutin PH, Hosobuchi Y, Phillips TL, Stupar TA (1981) Stereotactic interstitial irradiation for the treatment of brain tumors. Cancer Treat Rep 65(Suppl 2):103–106
58. Bernstein M, Cabantog A, Laperriere N, Leung P, Thomason C (1995) Brachytherapy for recurrent single brain metastasis. Can J Neurol Sci 22(1):13–16
59. Gutin PH, Prados MD, Phillips TL, Wara WM, Larson DA, Leibel SA, Sneed PK, Levin VA, Weaver KA, Silver P et al (1991) External irradiation followed by an interstitial high activity iodine-125 implant "boost" in the initial treatment of malignant gliomas: NCOG study 6G-82-2. Int J Radiat Oncol Biol Phys 21(3):601–606. doi:10.1016/0360-3016(91)90676-U
60. Laperriere NJ, Leung PM, McKenzie S, Milosevic M, Wong S, Glen J, Pintilie M, Bernstein M (1998) Randomized study of brachytherapy in the initial management of patients with malignant astrocytoma. Int J Radiat Oncol Biol Phys 41(5):1005–1011. doi:10.1016/S0360-3016(98)00159-X
61. Loeffler JS, Alexander E, Hochberg FH, Wen PY, Morris JH, Schoene WC, Siddon RL, Morse RH, Black PM (1990) Clinical patterns of failure following stereotactic interstitial irradiation for malignant gliomas. Int J Radiat Oncol Biol Phys 19(6):1455–1462
62. Prados MD, Gutin PH, Phillips TL, Wara WM, Sneed PK, Larson DA, Lamb SA, Ham B, Malec MK, Wilson CB (1992) Interstitial brachytherapy for newly diagnosed patients with malignant gliomas: the UCSF experience. Int J Radiat Oncol Biol Phys 24(4):593–597. doi:10.1016/0360-3016(92)90703-K
63. Hitchon PW, VanGilder JC, Wen BC, Jani S (1992) Brachytherapy for malignant recurrent and untreated gliomas. Stereotact Funct Neurosurg 59(1–4):174–178
64. Selker RG, Shapiro WR, Burger P, Blackwood MS, Arena VC, Gilder JC, Malkin MG, Mealey JJ, Jr, Neal JH, Olson J, Robertson JT, Barnett GH, Bloomfield S, Albright R, Hochberg FH, Hiesiger E, Green S (2002) The brain tumor cooperative group NIH trial 87-01: a randomized comparison of surgery, external radiotherapy, and carmustine versus surgery, interstitial radiotherapy boost, external radiation therapy, and carmustine. Neurosurgery 51(2):343–355 (discussion 355–347)
65. Gobitti C, Borsatti E, Arcicasa M, Roncadin M, Franchin G, Minatel E, Skrap M, Zanotti B, Tuniz F, Cimitan M, Capra E, Drigo A, Trovò MG (2011) Treatment of recurrent high-grade gliomas with GliaSite brachytherapy: a prospective mono-institutional Italian experience. Tumori 97(5):614–619. doi:10.1700/989.10721
66. Waters JD, Rose B, Gonda DD, Scanderbeg DJ, Russell M, Alksne JF, Murphy K, Carter BS, Lawson J, Chen CC (2013) Immediate post-operative brachytherapy prior to irradiation and temozolomide for newly diagnosed glioblastoma. J Neurooncol 113(3):467–477. doi:10.1007/s11060-013-1139-x
67. McLendon RE, Archer GE, Larsen RH, Akabani G, Bigner DD, Zalutsky MR (1999) Radiotoxicity of systemically administered 211At-labeled human/mouse chimeric monoclonal antibody: a long-term survival study with histologic analysis. Int J Radiat Oncol Biol Phys 45(2):491–499

68. Foulon CF, Bigner DD, Zalutsky MR (1999) Preparation and characterization of anti-tenascin monoclonal antibody-streptavidin conjugates for pretargeting applications. Bioconjug Chem 10(5):867–876
69. Akabani G, Cokgor I, Coleman RE, González Trotter D, Wong TZ, Friedman HS, Friedman AH, Garcia-Turner A, Herndon JE, DeLong D, McLendon RE, Zhao XG, Pegram CN, Provenzale JM, Bigner DD, Zalutsky MR (2000) Dosimetry and dose-response relationships in newly diagnosed patients with malignant gliomas treated with iodine-131-labeled anti-tenascin monoclonal antibody 81C6 therapy. Int J Radiat Oncol Biol Phys 46(4):947–958
70. Cokgor I, Akabani G, Kuan CT, Friedman HS, Friedman AH, Coleman RE, McLendon RE, Bigner SH, Zhao XG, Garcia-Turner AM, Pegram CN, Wikstrand CJ, Shafman TD, Herndon JE, Provenzale JM, Zalutsky MR, Bigner DD (2000) Phase I trial results of iodine-131-labeled antitenascin monoclonal antibody 81C6 treatment of patients with newly diagnosed malignant gliomas. J Clin Oncol 18(22):3862–3872
71. Reardon DA, Akabani G, Coleman RE, Friedman AH, Friedman HS, Herndon JE, Cokgor I, McLendon RE, Pegram CN, Provenzale JM, Quinn JA, Rich JN, Regalado LV, Sampson JH, Shafman TD, Wikstrand CJ, Wong TZ, Zhao X-G, Zalutsky MR, Bigner DD (2002) Phase II trial of murine (131)I-labeled antitenascin monoclonal antibody 81C6 administered into surgically created resection cavities of patients with newly diagnosed malignant gliomas. J Clin Oncol 20(5):1389–1397
72. Boskovitz A, Akabani GH, Pegram CN, Bigner DD, Zalutsky MR (2004) Human/murine chimeric 81C6 F(ab')(2) fragment: preclinical evaluation of a potential construct for the targeted radiotherapy of malignant glioma. Nucl Med Biol 31(3):345–355. doi:10.1016/j.nucmedbio.2003.10.008
73. Akabani G, Reardon DA, Coleman RE, Wong TZ, Metzler SD, Bowsher JE, Barboriak DP, Provenzale JM, Greer KL, DeLong D, Friedman HS, Friedman AH, Zhao X-G, Pegram CN, McLendon RE, Bigner DD, Zalutsky MR (2005) Dosimetry and radiographic analysis of 131I-labeled anti-tenascin 81C6 murine monoclonal antibody in newly diagnosed patients with malignant gliomas: a phase II study. J Nucl Med 46(6):1042–1051
74. Reardon DA, Akabani G, Coleman RE, Friedman AH, Friedman HS, Herndon JE, McLendon RE, Pegram CN, Provenzale JM, Quinn JA, Rich JN, Vredenburgh JJ, Desjardins A, Gururangan S, Guruangan S, Badruddoja M, Dowell JM, Wong TZ, Zhao X-G, Zalutsky MR, Bigner DD (2006) Salvage radioimmunotherapy with murine iodine-131-labeled antitenascin monoclonal antibody 81C6 for patients with recurrent primary and metastatic malignant brain tumors: phase II study results. J Clin Oncol 24(1):115–122. doi:10.1200/JCO.2005.03.4082
75. Sampson JH, Akabani G, Friedman AH, Bigner D, Kunwar S, Berger MS, Bankiewicz KS (2006) Comparison of intratumoral bolus injection and convection-enhanced delivery of radiolabeled antitenascin monoclonal antibodies. Neurosurg Focus 20(4):E14. doi:10.3171/foc.2006.20.4.9
76. Reardon DA, Quinn JA, Akabani G, Coleman RE, Friedman AH, Friedman HS, Herndon JE, McLendon RE, Pegram CN, Provenzale JM, Dowell JM, Rich JN, Vredenburgh JJ, Desjardins A, Sampson JH, Gururangan S, Wong TZ, Badruddoja MA, Zhao X-G, Bigner DD, Zalutsky MR (2006) Novel human IgG2b/murine chimeric antitenascin monoclonal antibody construct radiolabeled with 131I and administered into the surgically created resection cavity of patients with malignant glioma: phase I trial results. J Nucl Med 47(6):912–918
77. McLendon RE, Akabani G, Friedman HS, Reardon DA, Cleveland L, Cokgor I, Herndon JE, Wikstrand C, Boulton ST, Friedman AH, Bigner DD, Zalutsky MR (2007) Tumor resection cavity administered iodine-131-labeled antitenascin 81C6 radioimmunotherapy in patients with malignant glioma: neuropathology aspects. Nucl Med Biol 34(4):405–413. doi:10.1016/j.nucmedbio.2007.01.009
78. Zalutsky MR, Reardon DA, Akabani G, Coleman RE, Friedman AH, Friedman HS, McLendon RE, Wong TZ, Bigner DD (2008) Clinical experience with alpha-particle emitting 211At: treatment of recurrent brain tumor patients with 211At-labeled chimeric antitenascin monoclonal antibody 81C6. J Nucl Med 49(1):30–38. doi:10.2967/jnumed.107.046938

79. Reardon DA, Zalutsky MR, Akabani G, Coleman RE, Friedman AH, Herndon JE, McLendon RE, Pegram CN, Quinn JA, Rich JN, Vredenburgh JJ, Desjardins A, Guruangan S, Boulton S, Raynor RH, Dowell JM, Wong TZ, Zhao X-G, Friedman HS, Bigner DD (2008) A pilot study: 131I-antitenascin monoclonal antibody 81c6 to deliver a 44-Gy resection cavity boost. Neuro Oncol 10(2):182–189. doi:10.1215/15228517-2007-053
80. Larson DA, Gutin PH, Leibel SA, Phillips TL, Sneed PK, Wara WM (1990) Stereotaxic irradiation of brain tumors. Cancer 65(3 Suppl):792–799
81. Loeffler JS, Alexander E, Shea WM, Wen PY, Fine HA, Kooy HM, Black PM (1992) Radiosurgery as part of the initial management of patients with malignant gliomas. J Clin Oncol 10(9):1379–1385
82. Nwokedi EC, DiBiase SJ, Jabbour S, Herman J, Amin P, Chin LS (2002) Gamma knife stereotactic radiosurgery for patients with glioblastoma multiforme. Neurosurgery 50 (1):41–46 (discussion 46–47)
83. Souhami L, Scott C, Brachman D, Podgorsak E, Werner-Wasik M, Lustig R, Schultz C, Sause WT, Okunieff P, Buckner JC, Zamorano L, Mehta M, Curran W (2002) Randomized prospective comparison of stereotactic radiosurgery (SRS) followed by conventional radiotherapy (RT) with BCNU to RT with BCNU alone for selected patients with supratentorial glioblastoma multiforme (GBM): report of RTOG 93-05 Protocol. In: American society for therapeutic radiology and oncology 44th annual meeting, New Orleans, pp 94–95
84. Souhami L, Seiferheld W, Brachman D, Podgorsak EB, Werner-Wasik M, Lustig R, Schultz CJ, Sause W, Okunieff P, Buckner J, Zamorano L, Mehta MP, Curran WJ (2004) Randomized comparison of stereotactic radiosurgery followed by conventional radiotherapy with carmustine to conventional radiotherapy with carmustine for patients with glioblastoma multiforme: report of radiation therapy oncology group 93-05 protocol. Int J Radiat Oncol Biol Phys 60(3):853–860. doi:10.1016/j.ijrobp.2004.04.011
85. Tsien C, Moughan J, Michalski JM, Gilbert MR, Purdy J, Simpson J, Kresel JJ, Curran WJ, Diaz A, Mehta MP (2009) Phase i three-dimensional conformal radiation dose escalation study in newly diagnosed glioblastoma: radiation therapy oncology group trial 98-03. Int J Radiat Oncol Biol Phys 73(3):699–708. doi:10.1016/j.ijrobp.2008.05.034
86. Cardinale R, Won M, Choucair A, Gillin M, Chakravarti A, Schultz C, Souhami L, Chen A, Pham H, Mehta M (2006) A phase II trial of accelerated radiotherapy using weekly stereotactic conformal boost for supratentorial glioblastoma multiforme: RTOG 0023. Int J Radiat Oncol Biol Phys 65(5):1422–1428. doi:10.1016/j.ijrobp.2006.02.042
87. Curran WJ, Scott CB, Horton J, Nelson JS, Weinstein AS, Fischbach AJ, Chang CH, Rotman M, Asbell SO, Krisch RE (1993) Recursive partitioning analysis of prognostic factors in three radiation therapy oncology group malignant glioma trials. J Natl Cancer Inst 85 (9):704–710
88. Thames HD, Withers HR, Peters LJ, Fletcher GH (1982) Changes in early and late radiation responses with altered dose fractionation: implications for dose-survival relationships. Int J Radiat Oncol Biol Phys 8(2):219–226
89. Withers HR, Peters LJ, Thames HD, Fletcher GH (1982) Hyperfractionation. Int J Radiat Oncol Biol Phys 8(10):1807–1809
90. González DG, Menten J, Bosch DA, van der Schueren E, Troost D, Hulshof MC, Bernier J (1994) Accelerated radiotherapy in glioblastoma multiforme: a dose searching prospective study. Radiother Oncol 32(2):98–105
91. Werner-Wasik M, Scott CB, Nelson DF, Gaspar LE, Murray KJ, Fischbach JA, Nelson JS, Weinstein AS, Curran WJ (1996) Final report of a phase I/II trial of hyperfractionated and accelerated hyperfractionated radiation therapy with carmustine for adults with supratentorial malignant gliomas. Radiation therapy oncology group study 83-02. Cancer 77(8):1535–1543. doi:10.1002/(SICI)1097-0142(19960415)77:8<1535:AID-CNCR17>3.0.CO;2-0

92. Scott C, Curran W, Yung W, Scarantino C, Urtasun R, Movsas B, Jones C, Simpson J, Fischbach A, Petito C (1998) Long term results of RTOG 90-06: a randomized trial of hyperfractionated radiotherapy (RT) to 72.0 Gy and carmustine versus standard RT and carmustine for malignant glioma patients with emphasis on anaplastic astrocytoma (AA) patients. J Clin Oncol 384
93. Curran W, Scott C, Yung W, Scarantino C, Urtasun R, Movsas B, Jones C, Simpson J, Fischbach A, Petito C (1996) No survival benefit of hyperfractionated radiotherapy (RT) to 72.0 Gy and carmustine versus standard RT and carmustine for malignant glioma patients: preliminary results of RTOG 90-06. J Clin Oncol 15(Suppl):154
94. Fine HA, Dear KBG, Loeffler JS, Mc Black PL, Canellos GP (1993) Meta-analysis of radiation therapy with and without adjuvant chemotherapy for malignant gliomas in adults. Cancer 71(8):2585–2597. doi:10.1002/1097-0142(19930415)71:8%3C2585:AID-CNCR2820710825%3E3.0.CO;2-S
95. Stewart LA (2002) Chemotherapy in adult high-grade glioma: a systematic review and meta-analysis of individual patient data from 12 randomised trials. Lancet 359(9311):1011–1018
96. Stupp R, Dietrich PY, Ostermann Kraljevic S, Pica A, Maillard I, Maeder P, Meuli R, Janzer R, Pizzolato G, Miralbell R, Porchet F, Regli L, de Tribolet N, Mirimanoff RO, Leyvraz S (2002) Promising survival for patients with newly diagnosed glioblastoma multiforme treated with concomitant radiation plus temozolomide followed by adjuvant temozolomide. J Clin Oncol 20(5):1375–1382. doi:10.1200/JCO.20.5.1375
97. Stupp R, Mason WP, van den Bent MJ, Weller M, Fisher B, Taphoorn MJ, Belanger K, Brandes AA, Marosi C, Bogdahn U, Curschmann J, Janzer RC, Ludwin SK, Gorlia T, Allgeier A, Lacombe D, Cairncross JG, Eisenhauer E, Mirimanoff RO (2005) Radiotherapy plus concomitant and adjuvant temozolomide for glioblastoma. N Engl J Med 352 (10):987–996. doi:10.1056/NEJMoa043330
98. Laino C (2007) Glioblastoma: temozolomide + RT extends long-term survival. Oncology Times 29(23):16
99. Provencio M, Sánchez A, Garrido P, Valcárcel F (2010) New molecular targeted therapies integrated with radiation therapy in lung cancer. Clin Lung Cancer 11(2):91–97. doi:10.3816/CLC.2010.n.012
100. Gorski DH, Beckett MA, Jaskowiak NT, Calvin DP, Mauceri HJ, Salloum RM, Seetharam S, Koons A, Hari DM, Kufe DW, Weichselbaum RR (1999) Blockage of the vascular endothelial growth factor stress response increases the antitumor effects of ionizing radiation. Cancer Res 59(14):3374–3378
101. Hovinga KE, Shimizu F, Wang R, Panagiotakos G, Van Der Heijden M, Moayedpardazi H, Correia AS, Soulet D, Major T, Menon J, Tabar V (2010) Inhibition of notch signaling in glioblastoma targets cancer stem cells via an endothelial cell intermediate. Stem Cells 28 (6):1019–1029. doi:10.1002/stem.429
102. Levin VA, Bidaut L, Hou P, Kumar AJ, Wefel JS, Bekele BN, Prabhu S, Loghin M, Gilbert MR, Jackson EF (2010) Randomized double-blind placebo-controlled trial of bevacizumab therapy for radiation necrosis of the central nervous system. Int J Radiat Oncol Biol Phys. doi:10.1016/j.ijrobp.2009.12.061
103. Gonzalez J, Kumar AJ, Conrad CA, Levin VA (2007) Effect of bevacizumab on radiation necrosis of the brain. Int J Radiat Oncol Biol Phys 67(2):323–326. doi:10.1016/j.ijrobp.2006.10.010
104. Gutin PH, Iwamoto FM, Beal K, Mohile NA, Karimi S, Hou BL, Lymberis S, Yamada Y, Chang J, Abrey LE (2009) Safety and efficacy of bevacizumab with hypofractionated stereotactic irradiation for recurrent malignant gliomas. Int J Radiat Oncol Biol Phys 75 (1):156–163
105. Cuneo KC, Vredenburgh JJ, Sampson JH, Reardon DA, Desjardins A, Peters KB, Friedman HS, Willett CG, Kirkpatrick JP (2012) Safety and efficacy of stereotactic radiosurgery and adjuvant bevacizumab in patients with recurrent malignant gliomas. Int J Radiat Oncol Biol Phys 82(5):2018–2024. doi:10.1016/j.ijrobp.2010.12.074

106. Niyazi M, Ganswindt U, Schwarz SB, Kreth F-W, Tonn J-C, Geisler J, la Fougère C, Ertl L, Linn J, Siefert A, Belka C (2012) Irradiation and bevacizumab in high-grade glioma retreatment settings. Int J Radiat Oncol Biol Phys 82(1):67–76. doi:10.1016/j.ijrobp.2010.09.002
107. Hegi ME, Diserens A-C, Godard S, Dietrich P-Y, Regli L, Ostermann S, Otten P, Van Melle G, de Tribolet N, Stupp R (2004) Clinical trial substantiates the predictive value of O-6-methylguanine-DNA methyltransferase promoter methylation in glioblastoma patients treated with temozolomide. Clin Cancer Res 10(6):1871–1874
108. Hegi ME, Diserens A-C, Gorlia T, Hamou M-F, de Tribolet N, Weller M, Kros JM, Hainfellner JA, Mason W, Mariani L, Bromberg JEC, Hau P, Mirimanoff RO, Cairncross JG, Janzer RC, Stupp R (2005) MGMT gene silencing and benefit from temozolomide in glioblastoma. N Engl J Med 352(10):997–1003. doi:10.1056/NEJMoa043331
109. Lutterbach J, Weigel P, Guttenberger R, Hinkelbein W (1999) Accelerated hyperfractionated radiotherapy in 149 patients with glioblastoma multiforme. Radiother Oncol 53(1):49–52
110. Nieder C, Nestle U, Ketter R, Kolles H, Gentner SJ, Steudel WI, Schnabel K (1999) Hyperfractionated and accelerated-hyperfractionated radiotherapy for glioblastoma multiforme. Radiat Oncol Invest 7(1):36–41. doi:10.1002/(SICI)1520-6823(1999)7:1<36:AID-ROI5>3.0.CO;2-O
111. Prados MD, Wara WM, Sneed PK, McDermott M, Chang SM, Rabbitt J, Page M, Malec M, Davis RL, Gutin PH, Lamborn K, Wilson CB, Phillips TL, Larson DA (2001) Phase III trial of accelerated hyperfractionation with or without difluromethylornithine (DFMO) versus standard fractionated radiotherapy with or without DFMO for newly diagnosed patients with glioblastoma multiforme. Int J Radiat Oncol Biol Phys 49(1):71–77. doi:10.1016/S0360-3016(00)01458-9

Low-Grade Glioma

Priya Kumthekar, Jeffrey Raizer and Simran Singh

Abstract Low-grade gliomas are slower growing than their high-grade counterparts. They account for 10–20 % of all primary brain tumors. Median survival is between 4.7 and 9.8 years. The goal of treatment is to prolong overall survival while maintaining good quality of life (QOL). Recent data favors early surgical resection. EOR is associated with delayed tumor recurrence and improved survival. Additional therapy with chemotherapy or radiation is indicated in patients with high-risk features. Lower doses (between 45 and 50.4 Gy) have been shown to be as effective without adverse effects compared to higher doses. Recent trials have shown benefit in combining chemotherapy with radiation compared to radiation alone. The optimal chemotherapeutic regimen (PCV or temozolomide (TMZ)) remains unknown, although TMZ is easier to administer and better tolerated by patients. Novel molecular markers including 1p/19q chromosomal codeletion and isocitrate dehydrogenase 1 (IDH1) mutation have been correlated with treatment response and survival.

Keywords Low grade glioma · Chemotherapy · Radiation therapy · Surgery

Contents

P. Kumthekar (✉) · J. Raizer · S. Singh
Department of Neurology, Northwestern University, 710 North Lake Shore Drive, Abbott Hall, 11th Floor, Chicago, IL 60611, USA
e-mail: pkumthek@nmff.org

J. Raizer and A. Parsa (eds.), *Current Understanding and Treatment of Gliomas*, Cancer Treatment and Research 163, DOI 10.1007/978-3-319-12048-5_5

1 Introduction

Gliomas are primary central nervous system (CNS) tumors comprised of aberrantly growing glial cells, consisting primarily of astrocytes and oligodendrocytes. Gliomas are graded based on histological characteristics as outlined in the World Health Organization (WHO) into grades I–IV [1]. Grades I/II are categorized as low-grade gliomas (LGG) and grades III/IV are high-grade gliomas (HGG). LGGs are generally slower growing and account for approximately 10–20 % of all primary brain tumors [2]. The median survival time for patients with low-grade glioma has been shown to be between 4.7 and 9.8 years with a range of up to 13 years for certain subtypes [2]. Although LGG patients survive longer than those with HGG, the natural course for LGG is to undergo anaplastic conversion or dedifferentiation into HGG on average of about 4–5 years following diagnosis [3, 4]. The surgical and medical management of LGG has often been controversial in neurooncology; however, the uniform goal of treatment is to prolong overall survival (OS) while maintaining good quality of life. Treatment decisions for adults with low-grade glioma are determined by the presence of specific high risk characteristics. As we gain more insight into molecular and tumor markers, their impact on treatment will continue to evolve.

2 Prognostic Factors

LGG represent a heterogeneous group of tumors with various histologic subtypes (oligodendroglial vs. astrocytic), tumor markers (1p19q codeletions and IDH mutations), and clinical markers that can alter the outcome. Over time, prognostic scoring systems have been developed to guide treatment and patient care.

The EORTC trials 22844 and 22845 provided two distinct datasets allowing prognostic factors to be analyzed on one data set and validated on the other. The outcome was a set of validated high risk factors including: age over 40, astrocytoma histology, presence of neurologic deficits before surgery, tumor diameter of 6 cm or greater, and tumor crossing the midline. A favorable (low-risk) prognostic score was defined as two or less of the negative prognostic factors. A high-risk designation was given to patients with three or more of these high risk factors. Low-risk patients with two or fewer risk factors had an expected median survival of more than 7 years, but patients carrying three or more risk factors had a significantly shorter median survival time of 3.2 years [5].

Another prognostic scale was created from pooled data from the EORTC/RTOG and NCCTG clinical trials and analyzed to produce a prognostic scoring system. All patients included had central review of pathology to confirm LGG. Both PFS and OS were negatively influenced by worse baseline neurologic status, shorter time since first symptoms (<30 weeks), astrocytic histology, and a tumor size of >5 cm in diameter. In this study, age did not show prognostic importance. Based on this pooled data, prognostic calculators were created for clinicians to determine an individual patient's risk profile. The prognostic calculator can be found on the Internet at: http://www.eortc.be/tools/lggcalculator. A major limitation of this study was the absence of molecular data from the EORTC trials as this risk assessment was designed in the mid-1980s before they were widely available [6]. A third prognostic score was created by Chang et al. [7] who identified four preoperative prognostic factors in a series of 281 LGG patients. In this series, tumor size >4 cm, eloquent tumor location, age >50, and Karnofsky performance status (KPS) below 80 were found to be negatively predictive of OS. A scoring system was devised from these factors (range 0–4). The total score was inversely proportional to predicted survival. Such prognostic scoring sets identify high-risk patients who may benefit from adjuvant therapies postoperatively.

Of recent interest is the prognostic value of molecular markers in patients with LGGs. Hartmann et al. [8] sought to investigate various tumor markers found in LGG including p53 mutation, 1p/19q chromosomal codeletion, O6-methylguanylmethyltransferase (MGMT) promoter methylation, and isocitrate dehydrogenase 1 (IDH1) mutation for prognostic and treatment predictive properties. In this analysis, a total of 89 LGG patients were monitored without treatment following initial surgery, and another 50 patients received either RT or chemotherapy at upfront diagnosis. In both groups, the presence of 1p19q codeletion and IDH1 mutation were associated with prolonged PFS and OS in those who underwent treatment (either upfront or at progression). Other studies have also confirmed that patients with oligodendrogliomas, specifically those carrying the 1p/19q codeletion have a favorable prognosis and treatment response to both chemotherapy and radiation [2, 9, 10].

3 Surgery

Tissue is required to make the histological diagnosis of LGG. Although historically timing of tumor resection for LGG (upfront vs. delayed) had been debated, recent data favors early surgical resection for optimal survival outcomes [11]. Furthermore, both EOR and less volume of residual disease has been shown to delay tumor recurrence [12].

In the setting of severe mass effect, immediate surgery may be required. There are no randomized controls trials comparing early surgical intervention to observation alone and such trials are likely not feasible. Retrospectively, early resection has shown to improve outcomes for LGG patients. The largest such trial was conducted by Jakola et al. [11] and compared outcomes of LGG of patients from two separate hospitals who followed two separate surgical philosophies: early resection versus biopsy only for tissue diagnosis. There were 153 patients included in the study. At the institution favoring biopsy, 47 patients had a biopsy and 19 had initial resection. At the institution favoring initial resection, 12 patients had a biopsy and 75 had resection. At 7 years median follow up, median survival was 5.9 years at the center favoring biopsy and not yet reached at the center where initial resection was preferred. The patients treated at the institution favoring early resection showed improved survival compared to those at the institution that favored initial biopsy.

Eventually surgical intervention is inevitable in most patients [13] and a delay could lead to increased surgical morbidity and a decreased likelihood for gross total resection (GTR). Improved survival outcomes and delayed malignant transformation are seen with maximal safe surgical resections in LGG. Studies evaluating OS and PFS have uniformly shown improved outcome with EOR [3, 14, 15]. When possible, GTR should be attempted, although this may be limited by tumor location in eloquent cortex. Multiple retrospective studies have corroborated the benefit of greater EOR. Smith et al. [14] performed a retrospective, volumetric analysis of hemispheric LGGs in 216 patients and found patients with over 90 % resection showed a 5- and 8-years OS of 97 and 91 %, respectively; whereas patients with less than 90 % resection showed 5- and 8- years OS rates of 76 and 60 %, respectively. It should be noted there was no operative mortality and no significant association between extent of resection (EOR) and presence of new postoperative deficit ($p = 0.36$). Turkoglu et al. [3] conducted a retrospective study of 63 patients comparing the outcomes of those who had a GTR with those who had a subtotal resection (STR), partial resection, or biopsy. The findings from this study demonstrated that gross-total resection is associated with longer PFS ($p = 0.03$) and OS ($p = 0.04$) for patients with LGG on univariate but not multivariate analysis.

Shaw et al. [15] performed a prospective observation study of 111 adults <40 years old with low-grade glioma that underwent neurosurgeon-determined gross-total resection (GTR). The OS at 5 years was 93 % and PFS at 5 years was 48 %. Patients with residual tumor greater than 1 cm had a poorer PFS. Patients with over 2 cm residual disease had a subsequent 89 % recurrence rate. In comparison, patients with less than 1 cm residual disease had a 26 % recurrence rate. Of importance, this study demonstrated that adult LGG patients are not cured by surgery alone; there is greater than 50 % risk of tumor progression 5-years postoperatively. As such, patients with LGG warrant close clinical and radiographic follow up regardless of extent of resection.

Recently, surgeons have considered the possibility of a "supra-total" resection where patients have a resection beyond the borders of radiographic abnormality. Although controversial, Duffau [16] and colleagues have showed that "supra-total" resections of noneloquent left hemispheric LGG result in improved seizure outcome and safely delayed anaplastic transformation. Fifteen right-handed patients with a total of 17 tumors underwent resection of WHO grade II gliomas involving nonfunctional areas within the left dominant hemispheres. Awake surgery with intraoperative electrostimulation was performed in all cases. Supratotal resection involved removal until the surgeon reached cortical and subcortical areas crucial for brain function (i.e., eloquent language cortex). MR imaging showed that total resection was achieved in all 17 tumors and supratotal resection in 15. Despite transient neurologic worsening in 60 % of cases, all patients recovered and resumed normal life. Seizure control was obtained in all patients with a decrease of antiepileptic drug therapy. Median postoperative follow up was 35.7 months. Only 4 of 15 patients experienced recurrence (without anaplastic transformation).

These findings could support the use of awake surgery with functional mapping in the attempt to perform supratotal resection of LGG involving noneloquent areas in the left hemisphere. Because this study only involved 15 patients, further prospective trials are needed prior to considering this novel surgical approach as standard of care.

4 Radiation

Radiotherapy (RT) has been used in the treatment of LGG for several decades. Despite its long history in LGG, the optimal timing and dose of RT continue to be investigated (Table 1). Typically, radiation therapy is considered for patients after initial biopsy or resection for patients who are at a higher risk of early malignant transformation.

European Organization for Research and Treatment of Cancer (EORTC) 22844 and 22845 are two of the largest phase III trials ever completed in adult patients with LGG and they were designed to investigate optimal timing and dose of radiation. As mentioned previously, the EORTC 22844 and 22845 studies were used as a construction set for evaluating and validating high risk features, ultimately involving over 600 patients. A high-risk designation was given to patients with three or more high risk factors (age over 40, astrocytoma histology, presence of neurologic deficits before surgery, tumor diameter of 6 cm or greater, and tumor crossing the midline) [5]. This provided a guideline on which patients needed early intervention, namely radiation.

The EORTC 22,845 study compared early RT with delayed RT. After surgery, 314 patients were randomly assigned to early RT or deferred RT until the time of progression (control group). Median PFS was 5.3 years in the early RT group and 3.4 years in the control group. However, OS was similar between groups: median survival in the early RT group was 7.4 years compared with 7.2 years in the control group. Interestingly, at 1 year, seizures were better controlled in the early RT group. This study demonstrated that early RT after surgery lengthens PFS but does not affect OS [17].

Multiple studies looked at the optimal dose of RT with the goal to optimize tumor kill while minimizing both acute and long-term radiation toxicity. The largest such trial was the EORTC 22844 trial mentioned above. In this trial, patients were treated with either 45 Gy over 5 weeks or 59.4 Gy over 6.6 weeks with no significant difference in outcome observed between the two treatment groups. At 74 months follow up, the low dose arm had an OS 58 % and the high dose with an OS of 59 %. Furthermore, no difference was found in PFS between the two arms and QOL was worse in the high dose arm [18, 19].

A North Central Cancer Treatment Group (NCCTG)/RTOG/Eastern Cooperative Oncology Group (ECOG) study looked at over 200 LGG patients (with either astrocytoma or mixed oligoastrocytoma) treated with either low dose (50.4 Gy in 28 fractions) versus high-dose (64.8 Gy in 36 fractions) localized radiation therapy for

Table 1 Key studies in radiation and chemotherapy for low-grade glioma

Study	Design	No. of Patients	Radiation	Chemotherapy	Median follow up	PFS	OS
Karim et al. [18]	Prospective	379	45 Gy in 5 weeks	None	74 months	47 %	58 %
			59.4 Gy in 6.6 weeks			50 %	59 %
Van den Bent et al. [17]	Prospective	314	54 Gy Early	Variable, given to some patients at relapse		5.3 years	7.4 years
			54 Delayed until progression			3.4 years	7.2 years
Shaw et al. [20]	Prospective, Phase III	203	50.4 Gy	None	6.43 years		72 % at 5 years
			64.8 Gy				64 % at 5 years
Shaw et al. [24]	Prospective	251[a]	54 Gy	Radiation alone			7.8 years
			54 Gy	Radiation plus PCV			13.3 years
Pace et al. [28]	Prospective, Phase II	43	Variable[b]	TMZ at progression		39 % at 12 months	
Quinn et al. [31]	Prospective, Phase II	46	Variable[b]	TMZ at progression		Median PFS 22 months; 76 % at 12 months	
Hoang-Xuan et al. [27]	Prospective	60	None[c]	TMZ at progression	14 months	73.4 % at 12 months	
Kaloshi et al. [10]	Retrospective	149	None[c]	TMZ at progression	30.4 months	Median PFS 28 months; 79.5 % at 12 months	

[a] Total 251 patients were divided into high- and low-risk patients. High-risk defined as age over 40 and STR or biopsy. Low-risk patients were observed while high-risk patients were treated with radiation alone or radiation plus PCV
[b] Eligible patients were either newly diagnosed or previously treated with radiographic or clinical progression
[c] Eligible patients had no previous treatment except surgery and had radiographic or clinical progression

supratentorial low-grade glioma [20]. Survival at 5 years was not significantly different in the two RT doses (72 % with low-dose RT and 64 % with high-dose RT). This study confirmed the results of EORTC 22844 showing no OS benefit and a higher incidence of radiation necrosis in the high-dose RT arm.

5 Proton Therapy

Proton therapy is a novel technique that utilizes a heavier particle than standard photons to deliver radiation. Protons therefore enable dose reduction while sparing normal brain tissue during radiation given the lesser exit dose. There is limited data available for the efficacy of protons in adult LGG. Hauswald et al. [21] retrospectively analyzed patients with low-grade glioma (WHO grade I and II) treated with proton therapy. Proton beam therapy was administered to 19 patients total (median age 29). Median dose applied was 54 Gy in fractions of 1.8 Gy. Median follow up was only 5 months; therefore, PFS and OS data are incomplete. The treatment was tolerable with the most common complication of focal alopecia and fatigue. Further prospective trials with extended follow up are needed to determine the role of proton therapy in LGG treatment.

6 Chemotherapy

Much of the data for chemotherapy use in LGG has been extrapolated from data on the treatment of high-grade glioma (HGG). There is substantial overlap in the chemotherapeutic regimens utilized in HGG and LGG, which are most commonly TMZ and procarbazine/lomustine (CCNU)/vincristine (PCV). Chemotherapy can be given during radiation, adjuvantly following radiation treatment, or at progression. There is still controversy over the ideal chemotherapy agent, the ideal time of administration, and the optimal duration of chemotherapy treatment. Recent data suggests that chemotherapy can play a role in improving outcome of LGG patients (Table 1).

As the use of TMZ has become standard of care for HGG [22], its use in LGG has increased among the neurooncology community. Prior to the widespread use of TMZ, PCV was the chemotherapy of choice for gliomas and in long-term analysis of prior studies, PCV may still have superior survival outcomes specifically in codeleted gliomas [23]. However, part of this regimen requires intravenous administration and can produce significant hematopoietic toxicity for patients. TMZ is usually better tolerated and easier to administer compared to PCV. The efficacy of TMZ has never been compared head-to-head with PCV in a prospective, randomized trial.

The largest trial evaluating long-term benefit from chemotherapy in upfront LGG is the Radiation Therapy Oncology Group (RTOG) 9802 trial. In this study, a total of 251 patients with LGG were enrolled and divided into high-risk and low-risk LGG. Patients with favorable risk included those less than 40 years old and those with gross-total resection. Unfavorable risk patients were those over 40 years with STR or biopsy only. Patients in the favorable risk group were observed postoperatively. Patients in the unfavorable risk group were randomly assigned to RT alone or RT followed by PCV chemotherapy. A significant improvement in OS was noted for study participants who received PCV chemotherapy plus radiation (13.3 years median survival time) compared to those receiving radiation therapy alone (7.8 years median survival time) [24, 25]. This was similar to results seen in patients with grade III anaplastic oligodendroglioma and oligoastrocytoma who also showed improved response to treatment with PCV chemotherapy [26]. In addition, chromosome 1p/19q deletions have been associated with favorable radiographic response rates and prolonged survival in patients with anaplastic oligodendrogliomas receiving PCV therapy [27]. Loss of the heterozygosity of chromosomes 1p and 19q have been shown to be powerful predictors of survival and chemosensitivity in grade 3 oligodendroglial tumors [28] and presumably have the same prognostic and predictive impact in their LGG counterparts.

RTOG 9802 trial showed efficacy of chemotherapy in conjunction with RT. However, optimal timing of chemotherapy relative to radiation is unclear as is the best choice of chemotherapy. One study utilized neoadjuvant PCV in large unresectable low-grade gliomas or gliomatosis cerebri to avoid large field radiation. The median time to disease progression in newly diagnosed patients was >24 months [29]. Another RTOG trial (RTOG 0424) recruited high-risk LGG patients at upfront diagnosis for treatment consisting of concurrent radiation (54 Gy/30 fractions) and TMZ 75 mg/m^2 followed by 12 adjuvant cycles of TMZ 150–200 mg/m^2 for 5 days. Preliminary results are available. 136 patients were accrued. Median follow-up time is 4.1 years. Median survival time has not yet been reached. Three-year OS rate was 73.1 %, significantly improved from historical controls. Long-term data from this trial is still pending [30].

Multiple trials have evaluated TMZ in the recurrent LGG setting and have showed disease response. Pace et al. [28] prospectively examined 43 patients with LGG who were treated with TMZ (5 day on/23 off at a dose of 150–200 mg/m^2/day for 5 days per month) at the time of documented clinical and radiological progression. Median duration of response was 10 months with a PFS rate of 39 % at 12 months. Quinn et al. [31] conducted a phase II trial of TMZ (5 day on/23 off at a dose of 200 mg/m^2) for 46 patients with progressive low-grade glioma. The objective response rate was 61 %. Median PFS was 22 months. And lastly, Hoang-Xuan et al. [27] conducted a third prospective study of 60 patients with LGG and progressive disease on MRI treated with TMZ (5 day on/23 off at a dose of 200 mg/m^2) where objective radiologic response was 31 % and the median time to maximal tumor response was 12 months. Overall, there was a statistically significant positive correlation seen with the loss of chromosome 1p (with or without 19q deletion) and radiographic response to treatment. Retrospectively, Kaloshi et al. [10] examined 149 patients treated with TMZ (5 day on/23 off at a dose of 200 mg/m^2) in which 53 % experienced an objective response. The median time to maximal response was 12 months. The median PFS was 28 months. Combined 1p/19q codeletion was associated with a higher rate of response, longer PFS, and longer OS. All of the above studies utilizing TMZ in LGG treated patients with 10–14 cycles of monthly TMZ. In LGGs treated with TMZ, it has been suggested that prolonged duration of treatment (aka metronomic or dose-dense therapy) may achieve a prolonged response. Similar to their HGG counterparts, the methylation status of LGG may impact its response to TMZ as well [32, 33]. Metronomic TMZ has been tried in the LGG setting with the goal to overcome MGMT resistance in patients with newly diagnosed LGG. Kesari et al. [2, 34] looked at patients with LGG who received TMZ dosed at 75 mg/m^2 daily for 7 weeks followed by 4 weeks off treatment (11 week cycle). Treatment continued for a total of six cycles or until tumor progression and overall median PFS was 38 months. Molecular analysis revealed that patients who had a methylated MGMT promoter or deletion of either 1p or 19q chromosomes had longer OS. In LGG, dose-dense TMZ has not been compared to the conventional 5 day on/23 off regimen. However, in GBM patients, metronomic TMZ has been compared to the conventional "Stupp" regimen in the RTOG 0525 study which showed a lack of increased efficacy with dose-dense TMZ and increased toxicity for patients [35]. With the available data, the authors recommend using traditionally dosed adjuvant TMZ when indicated for 6–12 cycles.

7 Ongoing Studies

Current studies aim to further elucidate the timing of treatment, ideal chemotherapeutic agent and duration of therapy. Based on the long-term results of RTOG 9802 demonstrating improved outcomes with combined radiation and chemotherapy, the ECOG E3F05 phase III study of radiation therapy with or without TMZ for symptomatic or progressive low-grade gliomas was placed on hold due to a radiation only arm. The EORTC and the National Cancer Institute of Canada (NCIC) have joined forces to conduct a large Phase III trial comparing TMZ alone versus concurrently with radiation as first line therapy [2, 36].

Because of a possible superiority of PCV over TMZ, a trial comparing the beneficial effects of each chemotherapeutic regimen as well as their toxicities is of utmost importance [27]. Currently, there is a phase III intergroup study comparing TMZ and PCV for grade 3 anaplastic 1p/19q codeleted gliomas that is actively accruing patients [37]. Although this study population involves grade 3 gliomas, the results will be of great interest for the treatment of LGG patients.

Ongoing studies aim to evaluate TMZ both during and following radiation to assess for superior outcomes when compared to radiation alone in LGG patients. Other novel therapies including RAD001/everolimus (an mTOR inhibitor) [38] and autologous dendritic cell vaccines [39] are currently being investigated in the recurrent LGG setting for potential efficacy. Additionally, proton beam radiation is also being evaluated for safety and efficacy in adult LGG patients [40, 41]. The outcome of these studies may result in standard of care treatment options for both upfront and recurrent LGG.

8 Summary

Treatment of low-grade gliomas involves surgical resection, radiation, and chemotherapy. Maximal safe surgical resection is recommended at imaging detection to establish the diagnosis and to improve surgical and disease outcome. Studies have aimed to stratify patients into low- and high-risk categories to help guide the clinician in choosing which patients should be treated with postoperative radiation and chemotherapy versus observation only. Many retrospective analyses have concluded that postoperative RT is associated with prolonged survival. Early RT administered immediately postoperatively is associated with a longer PFS, but there was no significant benefit found for OS compared to delaying RT until progression. Therefore, the benefits of early RT such as improving seizure control must be weighed against the benefits of delaying RT. Delayed RT may be beneficial in cases of gliomatosis cerebri, utilizing neoadjuvant chemotherapy to shrink the radiation field. Higher doses of radiation have failed to demonstrate improved survival outcomes and can be associated with delayed toxicity.

Studies have validated the use of chemotherapy in combination with RT, although optimal timing, duration, and chemotherapy regimen is still being investigated. Long-term data from large studies have demonstrated benefit of PCV in addition to radiation; however, the use of PCV is associated with a high incidence of hematotoxicity and low tolerability. TMZ is a newer and better tolerated chemotherapy that shows efficacy in both the upfront and recurrent setting. Further investigation with direct comparison of PCV to TMZ is needed to determine which chemotherapeutic regimen is superior for LGG patients. Future studies will also aim to utilize tumor markers such as IDH, 1p19q codeletion, and MGMT in determining overall prognosis and best treatment options for each patient.

References

1. Louis DN, Ohgaki H, Wiestler OD, Cavenee WK, Burger PC, Jouvet A, Scheithauer BW, Kleihues P (2007) The 2007 WHO classification of tumours of the central nervous system. Acta Neuropathol 114(2):97–109. doi:10.1007/s00401-007-0243-4
2. Kesari S, Schiff D, Drappatz J, LaFrankie D, Doherty L, Macklin EA, Muzikansky A, Santagata S, Ligon KL, Norden AD, Ciampa A, Bradshaw J, Levy B, Radakovic G, Ramakrishna N, Black PM, Wen PY (2009) Phase II study of protracted daily temozolomide for low-grade gliomas in adults. Clin Cancer Res: Official J Am Assoc Cancer Res 15 (1):330–337. doi:10.1158/1078-0432.CCR-08-0888
3. Turkoglu E, Gurer B, Sanli AM, Dolgun H, Gurses L, Oral NA, Donmez T, Sekerci Z (2013) Clinical outcome of surgically treated low-grade gliomas: a retrospective analysis of a single institute. Clin Neurol Neurosurg 115(12):2508–2513. doi:10.1016/j.clineuro.2013.10.010
4. McCormack BM, Miller DC, Budzilovich GN, Voorhees GJ, Ransohoff J (1992) Treatment and survival of low-grade astrocytoma in adults–1977–1988. Neurosurgery 31(4):636–642 discussion 642
5. Pignatti F, van den Bent M, Curran D, Debruyne C, Sylvester R, Therasse P, Afra D, Cornu P, Bolla M, Vecht C, Karim AB (2002) European organization for R, treatment of cancer brain

tumor cooperative G, European organization for R, treatment of cancer radiotherapy cooperative G. Prognostic factors for survival in adult patients with cerebral low-grade glioma. J Clin Oncol: Official J Am Soc Clin Oncol 20(8):2076–2084

6. Gorlia T, Wu W, Wang M, Baumert BG, Mehta M, Buckner JC, Shaw E, Brown P, Stupp R, Galanis E, Lacombe D, van den Bent MJ (2013) New validated prognostic models and prognostic calculators in patients with low-grade gliomas diagnosed by central pathology review: a pooled analysis of EORTC/RTOG/NCCTG phase III clinical trials. Neuro-oncology 15(11):1568–1579. doi:10.1093/neuonc/not117
7. Chang EF, Smith JS, Chang SM, Lamborn KR, Prados MD, Butowski N, Barbaro NM, Parsa AT, Berger MS, McDermott MM (2008) Preoperative prognostic classification system for hemispheric low-grade gliomas in adults. J Neurosurg 109(5):817–824. doi:10.3171/JNS/2008/109/11/0817
8. Hartmann C, Hentschel B, Tatagiba M, Schramm J, Schnell O, Seidel C, Stein R, Reifenberger G, Pietsch T, von Deimling A, Loeffler M, Weller M, German Glioma N (2011) Molecular markers in low-grade gliomas: predictive or prognostic? Clin Cancer Res: Official J Am Assoc Cancer Res 17(13):4588–4599. doi:10.1158/1078-0432.CCR-10-3194
9. Baumert BG, Stupp R. European organization for R, treatment of cancer radiation oncology G, European organization for R, treatment of cancer brain tumor G (2008). Low-grade glioma: a challenge in therapeutic options: the role of radiotherapy. Ann Oncol: Official J Eur Soc Med Oncol/ESMO 19(Suppl 7):vii217–222. doi:10.1093/annonc/mdn434
10. Kaloshi G, Benouaich-Amiel A, Diakite F, Taillibert S, Lejeune J, Laigle-Donadey F, Renard MA, Iraqi W, Idbaih A, Paris S, Capelle L, Duffau H, Cornu P, Simon JM, Mokhtari K, Polivka M, Omuro A, Carpentier A, Sanson M, Delattre JY, Hoang-Xuan K (2007) Temozolomide for low-grade gliomas: predictive impact of 1p/19q loss on response and outcome. Neurology 68(21):1831–1836. doi:10.1212/01.wnl.0000262034.26310.a2
11. Jakola AS, Myrmel KS, Kloster R, Torp SH, Lindal S, Unsgard G, Solheim O (2012) Comparison of a strategy favoring early surgical resection vs a strategy favoring watchful waiting in low-grade gliomas. JAMA, J Am Med Assoc 308(18):1881–1888. doi:10.1001/jama.2012.12807
12. Berger MS, Deliganis AV, Dobbins J, Keles GE (1994) The effect of extent of resection on recurrence in patients with low grade cerebral hemisphere gliomas. Cancer 74(6):1784–1791
13. Recht LD, Lew R, Smith TW (1992) Suspected low-grade glioma: is deferring treatment safe? Ann Neurol 31(4):431–436. doi:10.1002/ana.410310413
14. Smith JS, Chang EF, Lamborn KR, Chang SM, Prados MD, Cha S, Tihan T, Vandenberg S, McDermott MW, Berger MS (2008) Role of extent of resection in the long-term outcome of low-grade hemispheric gliomas. J Clin Oncol: Official J Am Soc Clin Oncol 26(8):1338–1345. doi:10.1200/JCO.2007.13.9337
15. Shaw EG, Berkey B, Coons SW, Bullard D, Brachman D, Buckner JC, Stelzer KJ, Barger GR, Brown PD, Gilbert MR, Mehta M (2008) Recurrence following neurosurgeon-determined gross-total resection of adult supratentorial low-grade glioma: results of a prospective clinical trial. J Neurosurg 109(5):835–841. doi:10.3171/JNS/2008/109/11/0835
16. Duffau H (2011) Update on surgery for diffuse low-grade gliomas: brain mapping, hodotopy and neuroplasticity. Bulletin de l'Academie nationale de medecine 195(1):37–49 (discussion 49–51)
17. van den Bent MJ, Afra D, de Witte O, Ben Hassel M, Schraub S, Hoang-Xuan K, Malmstrom PO, Collette L, Pierart M, Mirimanoff R, Karim AB, Radiotherapy E, Brain Tumor G, the UKMRC (2005) Long-term efficacy of early versus delayed radiotherapy for low-grade astrocytoma and oligodendroglioma in adults: the EORTC 22845 randomised trial. Lancet 366 (9490):985–990. doi:10.1016/S0140-6736(05)67070-5
18. Karim AB, Maat B, Hatlevoll R, Menten J, Rutten EH, Thomas DG, Mascarenhas F, Horiot JC, Parvinen LM, van Reijn M, Jager JJ, Fabrini MG, van Alphen AM, Hamers HP, Gaspar L, Noordman E, Pierart M, van Glabbeke M (1996) A randomized trial on dose-response in radiation therapy of low-grade cerebral glioma: European Organization for Research and Treatment of Cancer (EORTC) Study 22844. Int J Radiat Oncol Biol Phys 36(3):549–556

19. Kiebert GM, Curran D, Aaronson NK, Bolla M, Menten J, Rutten EH, Nordman E, Silvestre ME, Pierart M, Karim AB (1998) Quality of life after radiation therapy of cerebral low-grade gliomas of the adult: results of a randomised phase III trial on dose response (EORTC trial 22844). EORTC Radiotherapy Co-operative Group. Eur J Cancer 34(12):1902–1909
20. Shaw E, Arusell R, Scheithauer B, O'Fallon J, O'Neill B, Dinapoli R, Nelson D, Earle J, Jones C, Cascino T, Nichols D, Ivnik R, Hellman R, Curran W, Abrams R (2002) Prospective randomized trial of low- versus high-dose radiation therapy in adults with supratentorial low-grade glioma: initial report of a North Central Cancer Treatment Group/Radiation Therapy Oncology Group/Eastern Cooperative Oncology Group study. J Clin Oncol: Official J Am Soc Clin Oncol 20(9):2267–2276
21. Hauswald H, Rieken S, Ecker S, Kessel KA, Herfarth K, Debus J, Combs SE (2012) First experiences in treatment of low-grade glioma grade I and II with proton therapy. Radiat Oncol 7:189. doi:10.1186/1748-717X-7-189
22. Stupp R, Mason WP, van den Bent MJ, Weller M, Fisher B, Taphoorn MJ, Belanger K, Brandes AA, Marosi C, Bogdahn U, Curschmann J, Janzer RC, Ludwin SK, Gorlia T, Allgeier A, Lacombe D, Cairncross JG, Eisenhauer E (2005) Mirimanoff RO, European organisation for R, treatment of cancer brain T, radiotherapy G, national cancer institute of Canada clinical trials G.radiotherapy plus concomitant and adjuvant temozolomide for glioblastoma. New Engl J Med 352(10):987–996. doi:10.1056/NEJMoa043330
23. Lassman AB, Iwamoto FM, Cloughesy TF, Aldape KD, Rivera AL, Eichler AF, Louis DN, Paleologos NA, Fisher BJ, Ashby LS, Cairncross JG, Roldan GB, Wen PY, Ligon KL, Schiff D, Robins HI, Rocque BG, Chamberlain MC, Mason WP, Weaver SA, Green RM, Kamar FG, Abrey LE, DeAngelis LM, Jhanwar SC, Rosenblum MK, Panageas KS (2011) International retrospective study of over 1000 adults with anaplastic oligodendroglial tumors. Neuro-oncol 13(6):649–659. doi:10.1093/neuonc/nor040
24. Shaw EG, Wang M, Coons SW, Brachman DG, Buckner JC, Stelzer KJ, Barger GR, Brown PD, Gilbert MR, Mehta MP (2012) Randomized trial of radiation therapy plus procarbazine, lomustine, and vincristine chemotherapy for supratentorial adult low-grade glioma: initial results of RTOG 9802. J Clin Oncol: Official J Am Soc Clin Oncol 30(25):3065–3070. doi:10.1200/JCO.2011.35.8598
25. RTOG 9802: A phase II study of observation in favorable low-grade glioma and a phase III study of radiation with or without PCV chemotherapy in unfavorable low-grade glioma (2014). http://wwwcancergov/newscenter/newsfromnci/2014/RTOG9802v
26. Cairncross G, Wang M, Shaw E, Jenkins R, Brachman D, Buckner J, Fink K, Souhami L, Laperriere N, Curran W, Mehta M (2013) Phase III trial of chemoradiotherapy for anaplastic oligodendroglioma: long-term results of RTOG 9402. J Clin Oncol: Official J Am Soc Clin Oncol 31(3):337–343. doi:10.1200/JCO.2012.43.2674
27. Hoang-Xuan K, Capelle L, Kujas M, Taillibert S, Duffau H, Lejeune J, Polivka M, Criniere E, Marie Y, Mokhtari K, Carpentier AF, Laigle F, Simon JM, Cornu P, Broet P, Sanson M, Delattre JY (2004) Temozolomide as initial treatment for adults with low-grade oligodendrogliomas or oligoastrocytomas and correlation with chromosome 1p deletions. J Clin Oncol: Official J Am Soc Clin Oncol 22(15):3133–3138. doi:10.1200/JCO.2004.10.169
28. Pace A, Vidiri A, Galie E, Carosi M, Telera S, Cianciulli AM, Canalini P, Giannarelli D, Jandolo B, Carapella CM (2003) Temozolomide chemotherapy for progressive low-grade glioma: clinical benefits and radiological response. Ann Oncol: Official J Eur Soc Med Oncol/ESMO 14(12):1722–1726
29. Stege EM, Kros JM, de Bruin HG, Enting RH, van Heuvel I, Looijenga LH, van der Rijt CD, Smitt PA, van den Bent MJ (2005) Successful treatment of low-grade oligodendroglial tumors with a chemotherapy regimen of procarbazine, lomustine, and vincristine. Cancer 103 (4):802–809. doi:10.1002/cncr.20828
30. Fisher BJ LJ, MacDonald DR, Lesser GJ, et al. (2013) A phase II study of a temozolomide-based chemoradiotherapy regimen for high-risk low-grade gliomas: preliminary results of RTOG 0424. J Clin Oncol 31 (suppl; abstr 2008)

31. Quinn JA, Reardon DA, Friedman AH, Rich JN, Sampson JH, Provenzale JM, McLendon RE, Gururangan S, Bigner DD, Herndon JE 2nd, Avgeropoulos N, Finlay J, Tourt-Uhlig S, Affronti ML, Evans B, Stafford-Fox V, Zaknoen S, Friedman HS (2003) Phase II trial of temozolomide in patients with progressive low-grade glioma. J Clin Oncol: Official J Am Soc Clin Oncol 21(4):646–651
32. Hegi ME, Diserens AC, Gorlia T, Hamou MF, de Tribolet N, Weller M, Kros JM, Hainfellner JA, Mason W, Mariani L, Bromberg JE, Hau P, Mirimanoff RO, Cairncross JG, Janzer RC, Stupp R (2005) MGMT gene silencing and benefit from temozolomide in glioblastoma. New Engl J Med 352(10):997–1003. doi:10.1056/NEJMoa043331
33. Everhard S, Kaloshi G, Criniere E, Benouaich-Amiel A, Lejeune J, Marie Y, Sanson M, Kujas M, Mokhtari K, Hoang-Xuan K, Delattre JY, Thillet J (2006) MGMT methylation: a marker of response to temozolomide in low-grade gliomas. Ann Neurol 60(6):740–743. doi:10.1002/ana.21044
34. Viaccoz A, Lekoubou A, Ducray F (2012) Chemotherapy in low-grade gliomas. Curr Opin Oncol 24(6):694–701. doi:10.1097/CCO.0b013e328357f503
35. Gilbert MR, Wang M, Aldape KD, Stupp R, Hegi ME, Jaeckle KA, Armstrong TS, Wefel JS, Won M, Blumenthal DT, Mahajan A, Schultz CJ, Erridge S, Baumert B, Hopkins KI, Tzuk-Shina T, Brown PD, Chakravarti A, Curran WJ Jr, Mehta MP (2013) Dose-dense temozolomide for newly diagnosed glioblastoma: a randomized phase III clinical trial. J Clin Oncol: Official J Am Soc Clin Oncol 31(32):4085–4091. doi:10.1200/JCO.2013.49.6968
36. Baumert B SR Radiation Therapy or temozolomide in treating patients with gliomas (NCT00182819)
37. KA J Radiation therapy with concomitant and adjuvant temozolomide or radiation therapy with adjuvant PCV or temozolomide alone in treating patients with anaplastic glioma (NCT00887146)
38. Chang S PM Phase II trial of RAD001 in patients with recurrent low grade glioma (NCT00823459)
39. Prins R Vaccine for patients with newly diagnosed or recurrent low-grade glioma (NCT01635283)
40. Lustig R Proton beam radiation therapy in treating patients with low grade gliomas (NCT01024907)
41. Ongoing studies Ref: http://www.clinicaltrials.gov/ct2/results?term=low+grade+glioma&pg=3

Treatment of Anaplastic Glioma

Wolfgang Wick, Benedikt Wiestler and Michael Platten

Abstract Anaplastic gliomas have received increasing attention over the past years. As opposed to glioblastoma, where the focus has been on the evaluation of novel compounds (with mainly disappointing results), in anaplastic gliomas relevant progress was generated with genotoxic therapies and translational work on biomarkers. Anaplastic gliomas are classified using single biomarkers, namely isocitrate dehydrogenase (IDH) or the related CpG island methylator phenotype (CIMP), alpha-thalassemia/mental retardation syndrome X-linked (ATRX), telomerase reverse transcriptase (TERT), p53, 1p/19q, and O^6-methylguanine DNA-methyltransferase (MGMT). With these molecular biomarkers, three main prognostically distinct groups have been defined: (i) CIMP-negative anaplastic gliomas, which have a similar prognosis as glioblastoma, (ii) CIMP-positive 1p/19q intact, and (iii) CIMP-positive 1p/19q codeleted gliomas. In the CIMP-negative, mainly *IDH* wild-type group, MGMT promoter methylation may be used to identify patients who benefit from alkylating chemotherapy. The mutually exclusive ATRX losses and 1p/19q codeletions are used to subcategorize anaplastic tumors with a mixed histology according to microscopic features. This eliminates the biological basis and clinical necessity for the diagnosis of mixed gliomas (anaplastic oligoastrocytomas). Retrospective long-term analysis of the EORTC 26951 and RTOG 9402 trials revealed that patients with tumors harboring 1p/19q codeletions benefit from addition of procarbazine, lomustine, and vincristine (PCV) chemotherapy to primary radiotherapy. RTOG 9402 suggests that this may be the case also for patients with 1p/19q intact tumors, but IDH mutation. Future developments in addition to the ongoing CATNON and CODEL trials, will focus on further refinement of the molecular predictors and development of treatments that not only increase survival but also maintain neurological function, cognition, and health-related quality of life.

W. Wick (✉) · B. Wiestler · M. Platten
Department of Neurooncology, Neurology Clinic & National Center for Tumor Diseases, University of Heidelberg and German Cancer Research Center, Neuenheimer Feld 400, 69120 Heidelberg, Germany
e-mail: wolfgang.wick@med.uni-heidelberg.de

J. Raizer and A. Parsa (eds.), *Current Understanding and Treatment of Gliomas*,
Cancer Treatment and Research 163, DOI 10.1007/978-3-319-12048-5_6

Keywords ATRX · Glioma · Brain tumor · Oligodendroglial tumor · IDH · MGMT · 1p/19q codeletion · Steroid · PCV · NOA · EORTC · RTOG · Temozolomide · Radiotherapy · CATNON · CODEL · CCNU · NDRG1 · 450k methylation arrays

Contents

1 Introduction

Over many years, most glial tumors have been considered mainly resistant to all genotoxic therapies. However, based on early trials radiotherapy has been considered a standard of care until recently.

1.1 Surgery

Despite the lack of a randomized trial or even a larger series focusing on anaplastic gliomas, there is a general agreement based on data derived from glioblastoma and low-grade glioma trials and patient series that patients with these tumors should undergo a maximal safe resection whenever possible. This statement is supported by the finding of a positive prognostic value of a macroscopic resection in most trials [1]. If a resection is not possible, a tissue diagnosis via open or stereotactic biopsy needs to be performed to allow for a detailed histological and molecular diagnosis [2].

Macroscopic resection also improves seizure control, particularly in patients with a long epileptic history and insular tumors [3]. In the European guidelines, the timing of surgery for oligodendroglioma is controversial in patients that are young, present with an isolated seizure (medically well controlled) and with small tumors [4]. Improvements in surgical techniques and imaging, together with enhanced treatment options for anaplastic oligodendrogliomas in modern practice, emphasize the importance of accurately determining a histopathological diagnosis as early as feasible.

1.2 Radiotherapy

Although radiotherapy (54–60 Gy, 1.8–2 Gy-fractions) has been considered standard of care for anaplastic oligodendroglial tumors, their chemosensitivity to nitrosoureas and temozolomide has long been recognized, and current data suggest that combination chemoradiation significantly prolongs survival, in comparison to radiation alone for grade III oligodendroglial tumors with 1p19q codeletions [4]. Patients treated with whole-brain radiotherapy have a higher incidence of leukoencephalopathy and cognitive deficits in comparison with patients treated with focal radiotherapy [5]. In studies using modern methods of radiotherapy a more limited impact on cognition is observed [6–8], although data related to patients who had more detailed neuropsychological follow-up at a mean of 12 years and were free of tumor progression suggest that those patients treated without radiotherapy maintain their cognitive status whereas patients receiving radiotherapy experience a decline in attention and executive functioning as well as information processing speed [9].

1.3 Chemotherapy

From the early 2000s, temozolomide chemotherapy had been developed as the standard of care for newly diagnosed glioblastoma [10], and as a therapeutic option for newly diagnosed low-grade [11] as well as anaplastic gliomas [12], as well as for salvage treatment of grade II–IV gliomas [13, 14]. Other options for patients with (progressive) gliomas include nitrosoureas like carmustine and lomustine. The latter is the most commonly used in control arms for modern trials for recurrent glioblastoma like the European Organization for Research and Treatment of Cancer (EORTC) trial 26101 (NCT 01290939) and is also a part of the PCV regimen.

Reports from the late 1980s noticed a greater chemosensitivity of many gliomas with oligodendroglial features (grade II and III oligoastrocytoma and oligodendroglioma) [15]. These reports have established PCV chemotherapy, which had been used since the late 1970s [16] for the treatment of malignant gliomas, as a widely accepted standard chemotherapy for many years. PCV chemotherapy usually consists of 4–6 cycles of 6 weeks with CCNU (lomustine) given at 110 mg/m^2 at day 1, procarbacine given at 60 mg/m^2 given at days 7–21, and vincristine given at 1.5 mg/m^2 i.v. (cap at 2 mg) on days 7 and 28. In clinical trials [12, 17, 18] this regimen has considerable toxicity, chiefly myelosuppression (CCNU and procarbacine), allergic reactions (procarbazine), and neuropathy (vincristine), but is very effective either as alone [12] or in combination/sequence with radiotherapy [17, 18]. With the introduction of temozolomide as a novel alkylating agent in gliomas chemotherapy options have expanded. As a single agent temozolomide is usually given on days 1–5 of 28-days cycles at a dose of 200 mg/m^2. Treatment duration is usually 8-12 cycles. Although there are no formal head-to-head comparisons in studies employing both, PCV and temozolomide, there were no differences in terms of efficacy [12]. It is widely accepted that the tolerability of temozolomide is better than PCV. Due to this reason and to optimize the efficacy of temozolomide, alternative dosing schedules have been developed and implemented in clinical trials including a weekly alternating schedule at 100–150 mg/m^2 [19] or in a 21/28-days schedule. While in the recurrent situation these intense dosing schedules have shown to be an option [20, 21], studies in primary glioblatoma have not indicated superiority over the conventional 5/28 days schedule [22] or deciphered a differential efficacy of the weekly alternating and the 21/28 days schedule [23].

The greater chemosensitivity of some glial tumors could, in part, be explained by *MGMT* promoter hypermethylation, but the 1p/19q codeletion and *isocitrate dehydrogenase* (*IDH*) mutations are also potential predictive biomarkers, though the mechanism of action remains elusive. It may well be that these "predictive biomarker" just signify a separate disease entity and not a molecular alteration for sensitivity towards genotoxic therapy. Furthermore, these and other molecular characteristics [13–16] may increasingly supplement the histopathology-based WHO classification and thus help to resolve the discrepancy between classification and clinical outcome.

This chapter on therapy for grade III glioma discusses (i) the molecular classification with its potential impact on therapy decision, (ii) data from randomized trials that guide the treatments currently used for patients with these tumors, and (iii) a pragmatic algorithm how to treat patients with anaplastic gliomas.

2 Molecular Biomarkers Separate Clinically and Biologically Relevant Groups of Anaplastic Glioma

Anaplastic gliomas can be robustly divided into three main molecular subgroups based on methylation and copy-number data independent of histology: CpG island methylator phenotype negative tumors (CIMP-) gliomas, which molecularly resemble mesenchymal, receptor tyrosine kinase (RTK) I or RTK II glioblastomas, non-codeleted-CIMP+ (non-CD-CIMP +) tumors with intact 1p/19q and CD-CIMP+ tumors with 1p/19q codeletion [24]. This classification provides a biologically and clinically more useful basis than the current WHO classification, which is based on histopathology alone. It also does not provide a basis for the diagnosis of a mixed anaplastic oligoastrocytoma. Here, *IDH*-mutated or CIMP+ tumors are either called a biological astrocytoma when they harbor an alpha-thalassemia/mental retardation syndrome X-linked (ATRX) loss (and mainly p53 mutation) or molecular oligodendroglioma when 1p/19q is codeleted (and often times a telomerase reverse transcriptase (TERT) mutated). In *IDH* wild-type tumors, the assessment of O^6-methylguanine DNA-methyltransferase (MGMT) promoter methylation status aids the decision whether or not to use alkylating chemotherapy [25]. A schematic overview on the current molecularly based subgrouping is provided in Fig. 1.

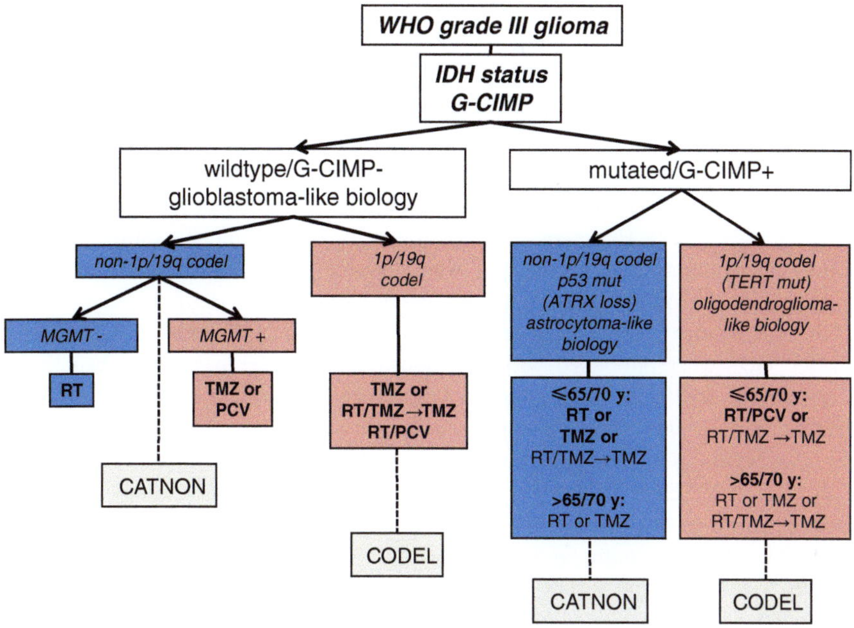

Fig. 1 A schematic overview on the current molecularly based subgrouping. In addition to the standard treatments, radiotherapy (*RT*), temozolomide (*TMZ*), procarbazine, lomustine and vincristine (*PCV*) or radiochemotherapy, there are trials for patients without 1p/19q co-deletion in the tumor tissue (*CATNON*) and with that molecular alteration (*CODEL*). isocitrate dehydrogenase (*IDH*), glioma CpG island hypermethylator phenotype (*G-CIMP*), radiotherapy (*RT*), temozolomide (*TMZ*), procarbazine (*PCV*), lomustine and vincristine, world health organization (*WHO*), years (*y*)

3 Lessons from RTOG 9802, EORTC 26951, and NOA-04/-08 Trials on Patients with Anaplastic Glioma

The most relevant development of the past decade is the delineation of patient groups who have a clinically meaningful response to chemotherapy. Radiographic response to chemotherapy has been reported in up to 70 % of newly diagnosed 1p/19q codeleted oligodendroglioma patients. In the 1990s, two randomized phase III studies for patients with anaplastic oligodendroglioma (AO)/anaplastic mixed oligoastrocytoma (AOA) (RTOG 9402 and EORTC 26951) and one trial in grade II gliomas (RTOG 9802) have been initiated to investigate the added value of PCV chemotherapy to radiotherapy. Another trial, conducted by the NOA (NOA-04) tried to establish monotherapy with temozolomide or PCV instead of radiotherapy in newly diagnosed anaplastic gliomas. In low-grade gliomas, the EORTC 22033 trial aimed to demonstrate superiority of primary temozolomide over radiotherapy.

The *initial reports* of the EORTC and RTOG studies in anaplastic gliomas, presented in 2006, concluded that there was no significant improvement in overall survival of patients with either codeleted or non-codeleted AO/AOA treated with either intense PCV followed by radiotherapy (RTOG 9402) or with radiotherapy followed by adjuvant PCV (EORTC 26951) (test arms) versus radiotherapy alone (control arm). Already in these final analyses, however, the progression-free survival of codeleted patients treated with the radiotherapy/PCV regimens was significantly longer than with radiotherapy alone [17, 18].

NOA-04 demonstrated that primary chemotherapy with PCV or temozolomide was as effective as primary radiotherapy both in terms of progression-free and overall survival [12]. However, all trials suffered from insufficient follow-up times at the time of the initial reporting and were not able to define the real impact or the appropriate subgroup of patients that benefited the most.

In 2012, more mature long-term survival data for both EORTC 26951 and RTOG 9402 were published which demonstrated an overall survival benefit for patients with 1p/19q codeleted tumors who received a combined radiochemotherapy: EORTC 26951 randomized 368 patients with newly diagnosed anaplastic oligodendroglial tumors to radiotherapy alone or radiotherapy followed by up to six cycles of PCV. Overall survival was 42.3 months with radiotherapy→PCV as opposed to 30 months with RT alone (HR = 0.75, 95 % CI 0.6–0.95). It was not reached versus 112 months in the radiotherapy→PCV versus radiotherapy arms for 1p/19q codeleted tumors (HR = 0.56, 95 % CI 0.31–1.03), but only 25 versus 21 months for non-codeleted tumors (HR = 0.83, 95 % CI 0.62–1.1). Although the addition of PCV significantly prolonged survival (HR = 0.75, 95 % CI 0.60–0.95) in the full trial cohort irrespective of molecular analysis, only the patients with the 1p/19q codeletion derived a clinically relevant OS benefit from the addition of PCV, especially when weighing toxicity of the combined treatment [26]. The data are similar for the North American trial. RTOG 9402 randomized 291 patients with newly diagnosed anaplastic oligodendroglial tumors to RT or RT preceded by up to four cycles of intense PCV. Overall survival was 4.6 years with PCV→RT and 4.7 years with radiotherapy alone (HR = 0.79, 95 % CI 0.6–1.04). Overall survival was 14.7 versus 7.3 years in the PCV→radiotherapy versus radiotherapy arms for 1p/19q codeleted tumors (HR = 0.59, 95 % CI 0.37–0.95), but only 2.6 versus 2.7 years for non-codeleted tumors (HR = 0.85, 95 % CI 0.58–1.23) [27].

Since the assessment of the 1p/19q codeletion does not identify all patients benefitting from radiochemotherapy with PCV in the RTOG 9402 trial, it was tested whether *IDH* mutations or a germ-line polymorphism, rs55705857, associated with *IDH* mutant gliomas identified the patients in RTOG 9402 who benefited from combined treatment.

This next retrospective subgroup analysis suggests that patients with 1p/19q codeleted and *IDH* mutated tumors (14.7 vs 6.8 years; HR, 0.49; 95 % CI, 0.28–0.85; $p = 0.01$) had the largest numerical benefit from combined radiotherapy and PCV. However, also patients with 1p/19q intact, but IDH mutated tumors showed a relevant benefit, when treated with radiochemotherapy versus radiotherapy alone (5.5 vs 3.3 years; HR, 0.56; 95 % CI, 0.32–0.99; $p < .05$) [33]. Both, the basis for this benefits, but the question why the EORTC 26951 trial did not suggest a predictive, but a merely prognostic role needs further workup and specifically confirmation by one of the ongoing or future trials in anaplastic gliomas.

Recently, another NOA trial on treatment of anaplastic astrocytoma and glioblastoma in elderly patients confirmed the value of a biomarker for treatment decisions in patients with anaplastic gliomas. The NOA-08 trial enrolled patients older than 65 years and a KPS $\geq$ 60. Patients were randomized to receive 100 mg/m^2 temozolomide given on days 1–7 and days 15–22 (1 week on/1 week off) of a 28 day cycle with the dose being adapted to the actual blood counts, or radiotherapy of 60 Gy administered in 30 fractions of 1.8–2.0 Gy. The primary endpoint was overall survival. The trial had a non-inferiority design. Of 584 patients screened, 412 patients were enrolled, and 373 patients received at least one dose of treatment and were included in the efficacy analyses. Median PFS did not differ between temozolomide [8.6 months (95 % CI, 7.3–10.2)] and radiotherapy arm [9.6 months (95 % CI, 8.2–10.8)] [19].

The value for MGMT status assessment for this group of patients was already suggested by the nonrandomized ANOCEF trial [28] and the retrospective analysis of the German Glioma Network [29]. The randomized NOA-08 [19] and Nordic trials [30] confirmed a predictive role of the *MGMT* promoter methylation status: In the NOA-08 trial, PFS and overall survival were longer in *MGMT* promoter-methylated patients who received temozolomide than in those who underwent radiotherapy (8.4 vs 4.6 months), whereas the opposite was true for patients with no methylation of the *MGMT* promoter (3.3 vs 4.6 months) [19]. In the Nordic trial, overall survival was longer in *MGMT*-methylated patients who received temozolomide than in those who underwent both radiotherapy regimens (9.7 vs 8.2 months), but similar for patients with no methylation of the *MGMT* promoter (6.8 vs 7.0 months) [30]. In general, methylation levels outside MGMT promoter methylation are rather low in the tumors of elderly patients and there is a poverty of common positive prognostic factors like IDH mutations [31].

The results from the long-term analyses of the RTOG and EORTC studies led to the suspension of enrolment into the NCCTG-led international intergroup phase III N0577 "CODEL" trial. CODEL was designed to address whether the addition of temozolomide to radiotherapy increased the survival of patients with codeleted tumors. After incorporation of the long-term data into the background of CODEL, the trial "Radiation Therapy With Concomitant and Adjuvant Temozolomide or Radiation Therapy With Adjuvant PCV or Temozolomide Alone in Treating Patients With Anaplastic Glioma"was amended in 2013 to answer the question whether progression-free survival of the combination of radiotherapy and temozolomide is not relevantly different from the combination of radiotherapy and PCV, but potentially harboring less long-term unwanted effects (NCT00887146). Despite its relevance given the general refusal to readopt the PCV regimen together with a lack of data to show that radiochemotherapy with temozolomide is just the same, the trial has not yet generated a momentum and accrual is slow.

At the same time, others are considering trials, in which radiochemotherapy with PCV as a standard is compared to chemotherapy (PCV or temozolomide) alone. Although the temozolomide alone arm of CODEL is designed to address this issue, specifically the timing and extent of neurocognitive health-related quality of life decline in these patients, it is not powered to reach conclusive results. The main focus of a current initiative of the NOA aiming at an international trial with the EORTC is to show superiority of temozolomide alone over partial brain radiotherapy followed by PCV in overall survival without functional deterioration.

Although it is intuitive to think that treating with temozolomide alone while postponing radiotherapy might delay cognitive decline, inferiority of temozolomide alone to the combined initial treatment, i.e., earlier tumor progression in the temozolomide alone arm, might produce the opposite results. Since neurocognitive decline has been shown to correlate with survival of glioma patients and often precedes radiographic progression [32], it is possible that patients treated with temozolomide alone might develop neurocognitive decline earlier than patients treated with radiochemotherapy. Hence, qualification by functional parameters of traditional efficacy endpoints, progression-free and overall survival, is one of the major developments of the upcoming trials. The other challenge is the identification and implementation of biomarkers not only as stratification factors or eligibility criteria in clinical trials, but also into daily clinical practice to determine which patients with a newly diagnosed or recurrent glioma should (or should not) be treated with chemotherapy.

The situation for patients with non-codeleted tumors is more complicated and less favorable. With respect to 1p/19q status, for non-codeleted patients combined radiochemotherapy is not the standard of care. The ongoing "Phase III Trial on Concurrent and Adjuvant Temozolomide Chemotherapy in Non-1p/19q Deleted Anaplastic Glioma: The CATNON Intergroup Trial."will show whether combined radiochemotherapy with temozolomide (concomitant and/or as an adjuvant maintenance treatment) is superior to radiotherapy alone (NCT00626990).

4 Algorithm for Treatment Decisions in Daily Clinical Practice

The basis for the need for testing 1p/19q, *MGMT,* and *IDH* status has already been discussed. In principle, standard of care for patients with an anaplastic oligodendroglial tumor with 1p/19q codeletion is (neo-) adjuvant treatment in addition to radiotherapy. Whether the chemotherapy regimen needs to be PCV or if temozolomide is a suitable alternative might be determined in the amended CODEL trial. Also, data for the exclusion of radiotherapy from the primary treatment may be generated from the long-term analysis of the NOA-04 trial or one of the new CODEL initiatives. Lastly, it is important to understand, whether the data from grade III oligodendroglial tumors can be applied to grade II and/or pure astrocytic tumors.

Recent epigenome-wide analysis, which also allow the determination of copy number aberrations allows classification of anaplastic gliomas into two main categories of G-CIMP+ and G-CIMP-negative tumors. A further subgrouping in the G-CIMP+ was based on 1p/19q status.

Tumor classification based on CIMP and 1p/19q status was significantly associated with survival allowing a better prediction of outcome than the current histopathological classification alone [24].

The data of Cairncross and colleagues on the long-term outcome of RTOG 9402 also justify the treatment of every patient with an *IDH* mutated oligodendroglial tumor with radiochemotherapy rather than radiotherapy alone [33]. *IDH* status is a better discriminator of outcome than histological grade in a pooled analysis of grade III and IV malignant gliomas, excluding oligodendroglial tumors [34]. Data from the NOA-04 trial and the German Glioma Network (GGN) demonstrated an interaction between *MGMT* and *IDH* status, and with that the basis for the need to test *MGMT* in patients with 1p/19q intact IDH wildtype tumors. The NOA/GGN analysis demonstrated that in patients with *IDH* mutations, there is similar benefit from initial RT or alkylating chemotherapy. In patients with *IDH* wild-type tumors on the other hand, a methylated *MGMT* promoter status is associated with superior outcome in patients treated with alkylating chemotherapy (with or without additional RT) compared to RT alone [25]. Hence, MGMT is predictive for response to alkylating chemotherapy only in the setting of an IDH1 wild-type glioma. MGMT may be bound and stabilized by factors like N-myc downstream regulated gene (NDRG)1, a central and druggable molecular hub downstream of epidermal growth factor receptor, and mammalian target of rapamycin. It integrates diverse therapy-induced microenvironmental factors to promote resistance toward alkylating chemotherapy. Besides hypoxia and radiotherapy, this is also the use of corticosteroids [35].

In addition to its classificatory relevance, determining gliomas biology, IDH mutated tumors may be a target for future demethylating or anti-IDH directed therapies, including decitabin (Dacogen®) (36) or AGI-5198 [36] or, if the most common IDH mutation R132H is present, specific active immunotherapy using peptides [37].

Other signatures and markers of different relevance were developed in the last years. A transcriptome-based retrospective analysis of samples from the EORTC 26951 trial demonstrated an improved outcome prediction when known molecular parameters where combined with transcriptome signatures [38]. Mutation/loss of *ATRX* in astrocytic tumors may not only serve as a positive prognostic factor, but also based on the mutual exclusivity of 1p/19q codeletion and ATRX alterations, a molecularly assisted classification for anaplastic gliomas may be suggested: In the NOA-04 trial, *IDH* mutant anaplastic astrocytoma and oligoastrocytoma without 1p/19q codeletion but with ATRX loss shared a similar clinical course irrespective of histology ("molecular anaplastic astrocytomas") as did anaplastic oligoastrocytoma with 1p/19q codeletion and oligodendroglioma ("molecular anaplastic oligodendroglioma"), leaving no room for the diagnosis of a mixed anaplastic oligoastrocytoma [39]. The above-mentioned 450k array epigenome-wide methylation analysis supports this concept [24]. The summarizing Figure shows the current status of biomarker testing essential to reach a biologically meaningful diagnosis, help with stratification for study entry and account for predictive factors to shape therapies for patients with these prognostically very heterogenous tumors.

5 Chapter Summary

- Chemotherapy alone with PCV or temozolomide is an option as primary treatment for oligodendroglial tumors.
- Recent long-term subgroup analyses of phase III trial reveal 1p/19q codeletion (and potentially also IDH mutations) as a predictive biomarker for combined (neo)adjuvant chemotherapy with PCV and radiotherapy.
- The value of 1p/19q most likely extents to non-oligodendroglial tumors.
- Molecular classification seems superior to classical histopathology.
- Relevance for nongrade III tumors remains to be shown.
- For 1p/19q intact tumors, IDH, and MGMT testing may be recommended.
- Mutated IDH is developed as a target for immunotherapy and IDH inhibitors and demethylating agents are tested in IDH-mutated tumors.

6 Key Terms and Definitions

- Isocitrate dehydrogenase: enzyme of the citrate cycle converting isocitrate to α-ketoglutarate by oxidative decarboxylation and are thereby involved in multiple metabolic processes. Mutations in the catalytic site at codon 132 function result in the inhibition of wild-type (wt) enzymatic activity and generate neomorphic neomorphic dominant enzymatic activity associated with the accumulation of the oncometabolite R-2-hydroxyglutarate.
- 1p/19q: Combined losses of genetic material from chromosomal arms 1p and 19q has long been recognized as a typical molecular signature of oligodendroglial tumors and has been shown to result from an unbalanced translocation which leads to the loss of one hybrid chromosome and thereby loss of heterozygosity. Recently, it was shown to be a predictive biomarker in anaplastic oligodendroglial tumors.
- MGMT: MGMT is a DNA repair protein that removes the alkylation of DNA induced by alkylating agent chemotherapy. An association of MGMT expression or activity and the benefit from alkylating agent chemotherapy in glioma patients has been observed for decades. Today, MGMT testing is done applying quantitative methylation-specific PCR, pyrosequencing or another method. Attempts are being made to introduce quality controls into the use of MGMT as biomarker.
- PCV: chemotherapy with procarbazine, lomustine, and vincristine that is used since the late 1970s for the treatment of malignant gliomas. PCV-Chemotherapy usually consists of 4–6 cycles of 6 weeks with CCNU (lomustin) given at 110 mg/m^2 at day 1, procarbacine given at 60 mg/m^2 given at days 7–21, and vincristine given at 1.5 mg/m^2 i.v. on days 7 and 28. It is now together with radiotherapy standard treatment for anaplastic gliomas with 1p/19q codeletion.

- Phase III anaplastic glioma trials: the EORTC 26951, RTOG 9402, and NOA-04 trials shaped our understanding on the biology of oligodendroglial tumors and their treatment.
- 450 k methylation arrays: allow methylation profiling and copy number analysis and with that classification of glioblastoma and anaplastic glioma into biologically and clinically meaningful subgroups.

7 Key Learning Points

- 1p/19q testing is a necessary part of good clinical care for patients with newly diagnosed anaplastic gliomas.
- Chemotherapy with PCV prior to or after radiotherapy is the current standard for anaplastic oligodendroglial tumors with 1p/19q codeletion.
- Presence of an IDH mutation in 1p/19q intact tumors allows to opt between radio and chemotherapy with temozolomide
- Absence of an IDH mutation should call for MGMT testing not to dismiss the need for alkylating chemotherapy.

References

1. Gorlia T, Delattre JY, Brandes AA et al (2013) New clinical, pathological and molecular prognostic models and calculators in patients with locally diagnosed anaplastic oligodendroglioma or oligoastrocytoma. A prognostic factor analysis of European Organisation for Research and Treatment of Cancer Brain Tumour Group Study 26951. Eur J Cancer 49:3477–3485
2. Olson JD, Riedel E, DeAngelis LM (2000) Long-term outcome of low-grade oligodendroglioma and mixed glioma. Neurology 54:1442–1448
3. Chang EF, Potts MB, Keles GE et al (2008) Seizure characteristics and control following resection in 332 patients with low-grade gliomas. J Neurosurg 108:227–235
4. Weller M, van den Bent M, Hopkins K, Tonn JC, Stupp R, Falini A, Cohen-Jonathan-Moyal E, Frappaz D, Henriksson R, Balana C, Chinot O, Ram Z, Reifenberger G, Soffietti R, Wick W (2014) European association for neuro-oncology (EANO) task force on malignant gliomaEANO guideline on the diagnosis and treatment of malignant glioma. Lancet Oncol 15(9):e395–403
5. Surma-aho O, Niemelä M, Vilkki J et al (2001) Adverse long-term effects of brain radiotherapy in adult low-grade glioma patients. Neurology 56:1285–1290
6. Taphoorn MJ, Schiphorst AK, Snoek FJ et al (1994) Cognitive functions and quality of life in patients with low-grade gliomas: the impact of radiotherapy. Ann Neurol 36:48–54
7. Klein M, Heimans JJ, Aaronson NK et al (2002) Effect of radiotherapy and other treatment-related factors on mid-term to long-term cognitive sequelae in low-grade gliomas: a comparative study. Lancet 360:1361–1368
8. Laack NN, Brown PD, Ivnik RJ et al (2005) North Central Cancer Treatment Group. Cognitive function after radiotherapy for supratentorial low-grade glioma: a North Central Cancer Treatment Group prospective study. Int J Radiat Oncol Biol Phys 63:1175–1183

9. Douw L, Klein M, Fagel SS et al (2009) Cognitive and radiological effects of radiotherapy in patients with low-grade glioma: long-term follow-up. Lancet Neurol 8:810–818
10. Stupp R, Mason WP, van den Bent MJ et al (2005) Radiotherapy plus concomitant and adjuvant temozolomide for patients with newly diagnosed glioblastoma. N Engl J Med 352:987–996
11. Baumert B, Mason WP, Ryan G et al (2013) Temozolomide chemotherapy vs. radiotherapy in molecularly characterized (1p loss) low-grade glioma. A randomized phase III Intergroup study by the EORTC/NCIC-CTG/TROG/MRC-CTU (EORTC study #22033-26033). J Clin Oncol 31, suppl; abstr 2007
12. Wick W, Hartmann C, Engel C et al (2009) NOA-04 Randomized Phase III Trial of Sequential Radiochemotherapy of Anaplastic Glioma With PCV or Temozolomide. J Clin Oncol 27:5874–5880
13. Yung WKA, Prados MD, Yaga-Tur R et al (1999) for the Temodal Brain Tumor Group. Multicenter phase II trial of temozolomide in patients with anaplastic astrocytoma or anaplastic oligoastrocytoma at first relapse. J Clin Oncol 17, 2762–2771
14. Yung WKA, Albright RE, Olson J et al (2000) A phase II study of temozolomide vs. procarbazine in patients with glioblastoma multiforme at first relapse. Br J Cancer 83:588–593
15. Cairncross JG, Macdonald DR (1988) Successful chemotherapy for recurrent malignant oligodendroglioma. Ann Neurol 23(4):360–364
16. Levin VA, Edwards MS, Wright DC, Seager ML, Schimberg TP, Townsend JJ, Wilson CB (1980) Modified procarbazine, CCNU, and vincristine (PCV 3) combination chemotherapy in the treatment of malignant brain tumors. Cancer Treat Rep 64(2–3):237–244
17. Van den Bent MJ, Carpentier AF, Brandes AA et al (2006) Adjuvant procarbazine, lomustine, and vincristine improves progression-free survival but not overall survival in newly diagnosed anaplastic oligodendrogliomas and oligoastrocytomas: a randomized European Organisation for Research and Treatment of Cancer. J Clin Oncol 24:2715–2722
18. Cairncross G, Berkey B, Shaw E et al (2006) Phase III trial of chemotherapy plus radiotherapy compared with radiotherapy alone for pure and mixed anaplastic oligodendroglioma: Intergroup Radiation Therapy Oncology Group Trial 9402. J Clin Oncol 24:2707–2714
19. Wick W, Platten M, Meisner C et al (2012) Chemotherapy versus radiotherapy for malignant astrocytoma in the elderly. Lancet Oncol. 13(7):707–715
20. Wick A et al (2007) Efficacy and tolerability of temozolomide in an one week on/one week off regimen in patients with recurrent glioma. J Clin Oncol 25:3357–3361
21. Perry JR et al (2010) Phase II trial of continuous dose-intense temozolomide in recurrent malignant glioma: RESCUE study. J Clin Oncol 28:2051–2057
22. Gilbert M, Mehta M, Aldape K et al (2011) RTOG 0525: A randomized phase III trial comparing standard adjuvant temozolomide with a dose-dense schedule in newly diagnosed glioblastoma. J Clin Oncol 29:2006
23. Tabatabai G, Wick W, Steinbach JP, Wick A, Schnell O, et al. *MGMT* promoter methylation as a prognostic biomarker for benefit from dose-intensified temozolomide rechallenge in progressive glioblastoma: First results from the randomized phase II DIRECTOR trial. J Clin Oncol Suppl Abstract 2015 (2014)
24. Wiestler B, Capper D, Sill M, et al. Integrated epigenetic and copy-number profiling identifies three clinically and biologically relevant groups of anaplastic gliomas
25. Wick W, Meisner C, Hentschel B et al (2013) IDH1 mutations determine the prognostic versus predictive value of MGMT promoter methylation in malignant gliomas. Neurology 81:1515–1522
26. van den Bent MJ, Brandes AA, Taphoorn MJB et al (2013) Adjuvant Procarbazine, Lomustine, and Vincristine Chemotherapy in Newly Diagnosed Anaplastic Oligodendroglioma: Long-Term Follow-Up of EORTC Brain Tumor Group Study 26951. J Clin Oncol 31:344–350
27. Cairncross G, Wang M, Shaw E et al (2013) Phase III Trial of Chemoradiotherapy for Anaplastic Oligodendroglioma: Long-Term Results of RTOG 9402. J Clin Oncol 31:337–343

28. Gállego Pérez-Larraya J, Ducray F, Chinot O et al. Temozolomide in elderly patients with newly diagnosed glioblastoma and poor performance status: an ANOCEF phase II trial. J Clin Oncol 2011 Aug 1;29(22):3050-5
29. Reifenberger G, Hentschel B, Felsberg J et al (2012) Predictive impact of MGMT promoter methylation in glioblastoma of the elderly. Int J Cancer 131(6):1342–1350
30. Malmström A, Grønberg BH, Marosi C et al (2012) Temozolomide versus standard 6-week radiotherapy versus hypofractionated radiotherapy in patients older than 60 years with glioblastoma: the Nordic randomised, phase 3 trial. Lancet Oncol 13(9):916–926
31. Wiestler B, Claus R, Hartlieb SA, Schliesser MG, Weiss EK, Hielscher T, Platten M, Dittmann LM, Meisner C, Felsberg J, Happold C, Simon M, Nikkhah G, Papsdorf K, Steinbach JP, Sabel M, Grimm C, Weichenhan D, Tews B, Reifenberger G, Capper D, Müller W, Plass C, Weller M, Wick W for the Neurooncology Working Group (NOA) of the German Cancer Society (2013) Malignant gliomas of elderly patients have a distinct molecular profile: an analysis of the NOA-08 study collective. Neurooncol 15(8):1017–1026
32. Johnson DR et al (2012) Early measures of cognitive function predict survival in patients with newly diagnosed glioblastoma. Neuro Oncol 14:808–816
33. Cairncross JG, Wang M, Jenkins RB, Shaw EG, Giannini C, Brachman DG, Buckner JC, Fink KL, Souhami L, Laperriere NJ, Huse JT, Mehta MP, Curran WJ Jr (2014) Benefit from procarbazine, lomustine, and vincristine in oligodendroglial tumors is associated with mutation of IDH. J Clin Oncol 32(8):783–790
34. Hartmann C, Hentschel B, Wick W et al (2010) Patients with IDH1 wild type anaplastic astrocytomas exhibit worse prognosis than IDH1-mutated glioblastomas, and IDH1 mutation status accounts for the unfavorable prognostic effect of higher age: implications for classification of gliomas. Acta Neuropathol 120:707–718
35. Weiler M, Blaes J, Pusch S et al (2014) The mTOR target NDRG1 confers MGMT-dependent resistance to alkylating chemotherapy. Proc Natl Acad Sci USA 111:409–414
36. Rohle D, Popovici-Muller J, Palaskas N, Turcan S, Grommes C et al (2013) An inhibitor of mutant IDH1 delays growth and promotes differentiation of glioma cells. Science 340 (6132):626–630
37. Schumacher T, Bunse L, Pusch S, Sahm F, Wiestler B, Quandt J, Menn O, Osswald M, Oezen I, Ott M, Keil M, Balss J, Rauschenbach K, Grabowska AK, Vogler I, Diekmann J, Trautwein N, Eichmüller S, Okun J, Stefanovic S, Riemer AB, Sahin U, Friese M, Beckhove P, von Deimling A, Wick W, Platten M (2014). A vaccine targeting mutant IDH1 induces antitumor immunity. Nature accepted
38. Erdem-Eraslan L, Gravendeel LA, de Rooi J et al (2013) Intrinsic molecular subtypes of glioma are prognostic and predict benefit from adjuvant procarbazine, lomustine, and vincristine chemotherapy in combination with other prognostic factors in anaplastic oligodendroglial brain tumors: a report from EORTC study 26951. J Clin Oncol 31 (3):328–336
39. Wiestler B, Capper D, Holland-Letz T et al (2013) ATRX loss refines the classification of anaplastic gliomas and identifies a subgroup of IDH mutant astrocytic tumors with better prognosis. Acta Neuropathol 126:443–451

Current Medical Treatment of Glioblastoma

Vyshak Alva Venur, David M. Peereboom and Manmeet S. Ahluwalia

Abstract Glioblastoma is the most common adult malignant primary brain tumor. Despite the advances in therapeutic options, survival of patients with glioblastoma remains dismal at 15–18 months. Current standard of care for newly diagnosed glioblastoma is maximal possible safe resection consistent with the preservation of neurologic function followed by concurrent temozolomide with radiation and adjuvant. Treatment options at recurrence include surgical resection with or without the placement of carmustine wafers, re-irradiation and chemotherapeutics such as nitrosoureas (lomustine, carmustine) or bevacizumab, a monoclonal antibody targeting vascular endothelial growth factor (VEGF).

Keywords Glioblastoma · Chemotherapy · Clinical trials · Angiogenesis · Targeted therapy

Contents

V.A. Venur · D.M. Peereboom · M.S. Ahluwalia (✉)
Burkhardt Brain Tumor and Neuro-Oncology Center, Neurological Institute,
Cleveland Clinic, 9500 Euclid Avenue, S73, Cleveland, OH 44195, USA
e-mail: ahluwam@ccf.org

D.M. Peereboom · M.S. Ahluwalia
Solid Tumor Oncology, Taussig Cancer Institute, Cleveland Clinic, Cleveland, USA

J. Raizer and A. Parsa (eds.), *Current Understanding and Treatment of Gliomas*,
Cancer Treatment and Research 163, DOI 10.1007/978-3-319-12048-5_7

1 Introduction

Medical therapies are an important component of treatment of glioblastoma. Adjuvant treatment of glioblastoma consists of temozolomide and radiation therapy. A number of cytotoxic and targeted agents are used in the therapy of recurrent glioblastoma. This review will focus on the role of the cytotoxic and targeted therapies in the management of glioblastoma.

2 Newly Diagnosed Glioblastoma

2.1 Cytotoxic Chemotherapy

A landmark international phase III trial established the role of temozolomide in the treatment of newly diagnosed GBM [1]. This trial randomized 573 patients with newly diagnosed GBM to receive either radiotherapy alone or radiotherapy and concomitant temozolomide followed by six cycles of adjuvant temozolomide. In the control group, patients received fractionated focal radiotherapy at 2 Gy per fraction 5 days per week, over 6 weeks, for a total dose of 60 Gy. In the experimental arm, patients received radiotherapy with concomitant temozolomide (75 mg/m^2 daily for 6 weeks). Patients then received up to six cycles of adjuvant temozolomide (150–200 mg/m^2 days 1–5, every 28 days). Two hundred and eighty six patients received radiotherapy alone while 287 received both radiotherapy and temozolomide. The median survival with radiotherapy plus temozolomide was 14.6 months compared to 12.1 months with radiotherapy alone. All patients in radiotherapy plus temozolomide group received prophylaxis for *Pneumocystis jiroveci* pneumonia with either inhaled pentamidine or oral sulfamethoxazole-trimethoprim during the concomitant phase. Grade 3–4 hematologic toxicity was noted in 7 % of patients during the concomitant phase and 14 % of patients in adjuvant phase. Fatigue was the most common nonhematologic adverse event. The 2-year survival in temozolomide plus radiotherapy group was 26 % whereas the radiotherapy alone group was 10 %. The survival advantage persisted at 5 years of follow up, 9.8 % in temozolomide group were alive at 5 years compared to 1.9 % in radiotherapy alone group [2].

A companion correlative study that evaluated tumor samples from 206 patients showed that methylation of the promoter region of the O^6-methylguanine DNA methyltransferase (MGMT) gene in the tumor was associated with superior survival [3]. O^6-methylguanine DNA methyltransferase removes the methyl group from the O6 position of guanine, reversing the cytotoxic effects of alkylating agents, making the tumor resistant to treatment. The methylation of the promoter region of MGMT results in inactivation of MGMT making the tumor more susceptible for damage by temozolomide therapy. Among MGMT-methylated patients, 5-year survival rate was 14 % in combined group compared to 5 % in radiotherapy alone group.

Recognizing that a different schedule of temozolomide may overcome chemotherapy resistance, alternative dosing schedules of temozolomide have been tried in the newly diagnosed glioblastoma [4]. A large phase III trial of 833 patients, RTOG 0525 was designed to test the efficacy of dose-dense temozolomide in newly diagnosed glioblastoma [5]. All patients received the standard concomitant phase of temozolomide and radiation for 6 weeks after initial surgical resection. In the adjuvant setting, the patients were randomized to standard adjuvant temozolomide or dose-dense temozolomide (75–100 mg/m^2 days 1–21, every 28 days). No statistically significant difference was seen in median PFS (5.5 months vs. 6.7 months) or OS (16.6 months vs. 14.9 months) in two arms. This trial confirmed the importance of MGMT methylation as a prognostic marker as it was associated with improved OS in both groups. There was increased grade 3/4 toxicity in dose-dense arm (53 %; $P < 0.001$), mostly lymphopenia and fatigue.

Strategies to increase the therapeutic ratio of temozolomide, such as the inhibition of DNA repair enzymes such as poly[ADP-ribose] polymerase [PARP] and base excision repair enzymes are being evaluated. These agents are being combined with radiation and chemotherapy to increase the cytotoxicity of the combination approach [6–8]. A cooperative group study of phase I/II study of iniparib, temozolomide, and radiotherapy in patients with newly diagnosed malignant glioma has completed accrual (NCT00687765). There is a planned Alliance study of veliparib and temozolomide following temozolomide and radiation in patients with newly diagnosed MGMT-methylated glioblastoma.

2.2 *Carmustine Polymer (Gliadel) Wafers*

The carmustine polymer wafer is a biodegradable matrix embedded with carmustine (bis-chloroethylnitrosourea) acting as extended release carrier system. Wafers are placed in the surgical cavity during tumor resection. They have been FDA approved for use in newly diagnosed and recurrent GBM during resection. They have not been compared directly with temozolomide in patients with newly diagnosed glioblastoma, and there are no data to support a clear survival advantage. A randomized trial compared carmustine polymer wafers to placebo in newly diagnosed high-grade gliomas [9]. Subgroup analysis showed median survival of 13.5 months in Gliadel wafers group compared to 11.4 months in placebo group in the 207 GBM patients; the difference was not statistically significant. Additional toxicities seen in the carmustine polymer group included cerebrospinal fluid (CSF) leak and intracranial hypertension (5 % vs. 1 % and 9 % vs. 2 % respectively) compared to placebo.

A recent observational study of 92 patients who underwent carmustine polymer wafers placement followed by concurrent chemoradiation with temozolomide reported a PFS and OS of 10.5 and 18.8 months, respectively [10]. Unclear if there is benefit of the addition of the carmustine wafer to standard chemoradiation.

2.3 Targeted Therapy

Angiogenesis is a highly regulated process necessary for new blood vessel formation and that occurs as a result of activation of a number of proangiogenic signaling pathways [11, 12]. Glioblastoma is one of the most vascularized tumors known, making antiangiogenic therapies a promising strategy [13, 14]. Glioblastoma is associated with a high degree of vascular proliferation [15, 16]. This results in upregulation of proangiogenic factors such vascular endothelial growth factor (VEGF), fibroblast growth factor (FGF), and platelet-derived growth factor (PDGF) [13]. Increased expression of VEGF in GBM correlates with increased tumor aggressiveness and poor survival [17]. Bevacizumab is a humanized monoclonal antibody that binds to the ligand VEGF-A, and the inhibition of the VEGF normalizes the vasculature of gliomas [18].

Two large randomized phase III trials (RTOG 0825 [19] and AVAglio [20]) examined the efficacy of bevacizumab in combination with radiation and temozolomide in patients with newly diagnosed GBM. In RTOG 0825, 637 patients were randomized to standard temozolomide and radiotherapy (control group-placebo) or bevacizumab in addition to standard temozolomide and radiotherapy (experimental group) [19]. Although PFS was increased in the bevacizumab arm (11 months vs. 7.3 months, $p = 0.004$), the improvement did not meet the prespecified criteria for a positive study. No difference was found between the two arms for OS (both 16 months). Patients with MGMT methylation had superior PFS and OS ($p < 0.001$). Neither the 9-gene signature nor MGMT predicted selective benefit for bevacizumab treatment, but best prognosis patients (MGMT methylation, favorable 9-gene) had a worse survival trend with bevacizumab (16 months vs. 25 months, $p = 0.08$). The study identified the PRO GBM panel as a gene signature that predicted for benefit with bevacizumab. However, this needs to be validated in prospective trial. Increased grade ≥3 toxicity was seen with bevacizumab group, mostly neutropenia, hypertension, and thrombo-embolic disease. Results of a quality of life analysis favored the chemoradiation alone group. Patients who underwent a biopsy were excluded from the trial due to the requirement of tissue for correlative studies, a group that may derive the most benefit with treatment with bevacizumab.

In the AVAglio study (Roche/Genentech sponsored), 921 patients were randomized to receive bevacizumab or placebo in combination with radiation and temozolomide. The addition of bevacizumab to radiation and temozolomide significantly prolonged PFS (HR 0.64, $p < 0.0001$; median 10.6 months vs. 6.2 months) as compared to radiation and temozolomide [20]. However, the addition of bevacizumab did not improve OS (16.8 months vs. 16.7 months, HR 0.88, $p = 0.1$). In this study, the patients treated on the experimental arm showed improved quality of life as measured by five scales of the QLQ-C30 and BN20 survey instruments. The patients treated on the experimental had longer time off from steroids and maintained their performance status longer as compared to the control group.

Patients with unmethylated MGMT glioblastoma have inferior outcomes as compared to those with MGMT-methylated glioblastoma and temozolomide is less effective in these patients. Hence the GLARIUS trial eliminated the temozolomide in the experimental arm. In a phase II trial, 170 patients with unmethylated MGMT glioblastoma were randomized to bevacizumab with radiotherapy followed by maintenance bevacizumab and irinotecan (experimental arm) compared to standard temozolomide during radiation followed by 6 cycles of temozolomide (control arm) [21]. The progression-free survival at 6 months (primary endpoint) in experimental arm was superior (72 % vs. 26 %).

Cilengitide (EMD121974), an integrin inhibitor that showed some promise in recurrent glioblastoma [22, 23], was evaluated in newly diagnosed glioblastoma trials. In the CENTRIC study, 545 patients with newly diagnosed glioblastoma with MGMT promoter methylation were randomized to cilengitide in addition to standard radiation and temozolomide [24]. The overall survival was similar in both arms (26 months vs. 26 months), and the study did not show any additional benefit with cilengitide in this patient population [24]. The CORE trial, a three-arm multicenter phase II trial, randomized patients with unmethylated MGMT glioblastoma to standard (2 times a week) or intensive (5 times a week) cilengitide in addition to radiation and temozolomide compared to standard therapy of radiation and temozolomide (control group) [25]. There was suggestion of benefit of cilengitide with median OS of 16 months in the standard dose of cilengitide arm compared to the median OS was 13 months in the control group (HR 0.69; $p = 0.033$). However, this drug is not being further developed.

2.4 Summary and Recommendation

For newly diagnosed glioblastoma, we recommend participation in a clinical trial. In case the patient is not eligible for a clinical trial and has good performance status, we use 6 weeks of concurrent radiotherapy (60 Gy in 30 fractions) with daily temozolomide (75 mg/m^2) followed by adjuvant temozolomide (150–200 mg/m^2 day 1–5 every 28 days) for 6 cycles (level 1 evidence). It reasonable alternative to use up to 12 cycles however no trials have compared 12 versus 6 cycles; RTOG 0525 suggested a benefit for 12 months but the number were heavily weighted for patients who received 12 months of therapy so hard to interpret. For post-radiation temozolomide, dose-dense therapy did not show an advantage over the standard 5/28 day approach (Level 1 evidence). We prefer not to use adjuvant nitrosoureas or carmustine polymer wafers (often exclusion criteria for clinical trial participation).

3 Recurrent Glioblastoma

Treatment options for recurrent GBM must be tailored to the individual. Few agents have proven activity.

3.1 Cytotoxic Chemotherapy

For patients who recur after initial treatment with temozolomide and who are not candidates for a clinical trial and have with small tumors that are not very symptomatic, nitrosoureas or nitrosoureas containing regimen is a reasonable approach. Nitrosoureas such as lomustine, carmustine either as single agents or in combination —procarbazine, lomustine, and vincristine (PCV regimen) are commonly used in United States.

In a phase II study of 40 with recurrent glioblastoma patients treated with carmustine (BCNU) following surgery and standard radiotherapy, a median time to progression (TTP) of 13 weeks was noted [26]. Progression-free survival at 6 months was 17 %. Response to chemotherapy was a significant prognostic factor for TTP on multivariate analysis.

Two phase III trials of enzastaurin and cediranib used single-agent lomustine as the control arm [27, 28]. In the enzastaurin phase II trial, median PFS, PFS-6, and OS of 1.6, 19 %, and 7.1 months respectively were seen in the recurrent glioblastoma patients in the lomustine arm [27]. In the phase III trial that examined the efficacy of cediranib, the median PFS and OS with lomustine were 2.7 and 9.8 months, respectively [28]. Based on these data from these two large phase III trials, there has been renewed interest in using lomustine in the patients with recurrent glioblastoma who are not eligible for clinical trial or in whom bevacizumab is a not a preferred option.

A trial of 86 patients with recurrent glioblastoma evaluated procarbazine, lomustine, and vincristine (PCV) [29]. Median PFS of 17 weeks and PFS-6 of 38 % was seen and 3 patients achieved partial responses (PR). World Health Organization grade 3/4 hematologic toxicity of 26 % was the most common side effect noted on this study. Many investigators, however, do not use the PCV regimen in favor of single-agent lomustine due to the increased toxicity of the combination and the lack of blood–brain barrier penetration of vincristine.

Dose-dense or dose-intense or metronomic temozolomide has been evaluated in number of phase II studies of patients with recurrent malignant glioma [30–33]. In RESCUE study, a phase II study of recurrent malignant glioma, 120 patients were treated with continuous daily temozolomide, 50 mg/m^2/day [32]. 6-month progression-free survival (PFS-6) of 24 % was seen in the recurrent glioblastoma group.

3.2 Carmustine Polymer (Gliadel) Wafers

A phase III trial in the setting of recurrent high-grade gliomas enrolled 227 patients of which 145 had GBM [34]. The 6-month survival was 50 % greater in those implanted with Gliadel wafers as compared to placebo. Major adverse effects noted included seizures, cerebral edema, and intracranial infections. Given the heterogeneous patient population in this report, the role of carmustine wafers for any specific high-grade glioma histology is difficult to discern.

3.3 Targeted Therapies

The earliest report of bevacizumab use was from Dr. Stark-Vance, who treated 21 patients with recurrent high-grade glioma, including 11 patients with glioblastoma, with bevacizumab and irinotecan [35]. There were one complete response (CR), 8 PR, and 11 stable diseases (SD). The overall response rate (ORR) was 43 %.

The majority of initial clinical trials in high-grade gliomas utilized bevacizumab in combination with irinotecan based on the original combination regimen used in colorectal cancer. A phase II trial of 35 patients with recurrent glioblastoma evaluated bevacizumab and irinotecan [36]. The PFS-6 of 46 % and OS of 9.7 months led to a larger multicenter prospective randomized noncomparative trial, the BRAIN study [37]. In this study, 167 recurrent glioblastoma patients were randomized to treatment with bevacizumab with or without irinotecan. Overall response rates (ORR) of 38 % versus 28 %, PFS-6 of 50 % versus 46 %, and OS of 8.7 months versus 9.2 months were seen in the combination and bevacizumab alone arm, respectively. This trial showed improved PFS-6 and ORR compared to historical controls. Bevacizumab use was associated with a steroid sparing effect. In the NCI 06-C-0064E phase II trial, 48 patients with recurrent glioblastoma were treated with bevacizumab monotherapy, and received irinotecan at progression [38]. In this study, ORR of 35 % and PFS-6 of 29 % was noted, and there was no benefit of adding irinotecan at progression. Based on the ORR seen in the BRAIN trial and NCI 06-C-0064E trials, bevacizumab received the US FDA accelerated provisional approval in recurrent glioblastoma [37, 38]. However, the European regulatory authority did not approve bevacizumab for use in recurrent glioblastoma due to the lack of a control arm in these two trials.

Multiple chemotherapy or targeted agents have undergone extensive evaluation in combination with bevacizumab, primarily in recurrent glioblastoma. These include combination with etoposide [39], carboplatin [40], temozolomide [41] or alternative dosing [42] or lower dose [43]. The results of these studies have been comparable to the bevacizumab arm of the BRAIN study.

Two randomized phase II trials have evaluated the benefit of chemotherapy to bevacizumab. A phase II trial (CABARET) randomized patients to treatment with bevacizumab with or without carboplatin. The PFS-6 of 26 % and OS of 6.9 months for the combination were similar to PFS-6 of 24 % and OS of 6.4 months observed for bevacizumab monotherapy [28]. In the BELOB study, a Dutch three-arm multicenter randomized phase II study, 148 recurrent glioblastoma patients were randomized to bevacizumab, lomustine, or the combination of bevacizumab and lomustine. The PFS-6 was 16, 13, and 41 %, and the OS at 9 months was 38, 43, and 59 %, respectively [44]. The combination of bevacizumab and lomustine met the prespecified primary endpoint of OS at 9 months of 55 % and is undergoing evaluation in phase III study, EORTC (NCT01290939). Interestingly, the single-agent arm did far worse than other trials.

A number of agents targeting VEGF have been examined. Cediranib (AZD2171), an orally administered pan-VEGF receptor inhibitor, showed promising results in a

Table 1 Randomized trials in newly diagnosed glioblastoma with medical therapies (last decade)

Study (reference)	Number of patients	Treatment arms	PFS (months)	OS (months)	Comments
EORTC/NCI [1]	573	RT/TMZ versus RT	6.9 versus 5.0	15 versus 12	RT/TMZ superior to RT alone
RTOG 0525 [5]	833	Standard dose TMZ (days 1–5 every 28 days) versus dose-dense TMZ (days 1–21 every 28 days)	5.5 versus 6.7	17 versus 15	No significant improvement in OS or PFS with dose-dense TMZ/RT
RTOG 0825 [19]	637	RT/TMZ/Bev versus RT/TMZ	11 versus 7.3	16 versus 16	PFS longer in Bev group; no significant difference in OS
AVAGLIO [20]	921	RT/TMZ/Bev versus RT/TMZ	11 versus 6.2	17 versus 17	PFS longer in Bev group; no significant difference in OS
GLARIUS [21]	170	RT/TMZ/Bev + Bev/Iri[a] versus RT/TMZ	9.7 versus 6.0	17 versus 15	PFS-6 in Bev/Iri arm superior unmethylated MGMT GBM
CENTRIC [24]	545	RT/TMZ/CIL versus RT/TMZ	13 versus 11	26 versus 26	CIL did not prolong PFS or OS in methylated MGMT GBM
CORE [25]	265	RT/TMZ/CIL_2 versus RT/TMZ/CIL_5 versus RT/TMZ	5.6 versus 5.9 versus 4.1	16 versus 14 versus 13	Median OS increased with addition of CIL_2 but not with CIL_5 in unmethylated MGMT GBM

RT/TMZ-radiation with concurrent temozolomide followed by adjuvant temozolomide; *PFS* progression-free survival; *PFS* 6-progression-free survival at 6 months; *OS* overall survival; *RT* radiation therapy; *TMZ* temozolomide; *Bev* bevacizumab; *Iri* irinotecan; *MGMT* O^6 -methylguanine DNA methyltransferase; *CIL* cilengitide; CIL_2 cilengitide 2 times/week (standard dose); CIL_5 cilengitide 5 times/week (dose intense)

[a] Bev/Iri substituted for adjuvant temozolomide

Table 2 Randomized trials in recurrent glioblastoma with medical therapies (last decade)

Study (reference)	Number of patients	Treatment	PFS (months)	OS (months)	Comments
Bev versus Bev/Iri [35]	167	Bev versus Bev/Iri	46 % versus 50 %[a]	9.2 versus 8.7	No advantage to addition of irinotecan
Enzastaurin versus Lomustine [27]	266	Enzastaurin versus lomustine	1.5 versus 1.6	6.6 versus 7.1	PFS, OS not superior
REGAL [46]	325	Cediranib versus lomustine versus cediranib/lomustine	92 versus 82 versus 125 days	8.0 versus 9.8 versus 9.4	Cediranib-containing arms not superior to lomustine
CABARET [28]	122	Bev/Carboplatin versus Bev	26 % versus 24 %[a]	6.9 versus 6.4	Bev/Carboplatin not superior
BELOB [44]	140	Bev versus Lomustine versus Bev/Lomustine	3 versus 2 versus 4	38 % versus 43 % versus 59 %[b]	Bev/lomustine met primary endpoint of OS at 9 months (55 %). Phase III bev/lomustine versus lomustine ongoing

PFS progression-free survival; *OS* overall survival; *Bev* bevacizumab
[a] PFS_6 (PFS at 6 months)

single-center phase II study [45]. However, the phase III randomized trial did not show a statistical improvement in PFS with cediranib either as monotherapy or in combination with lomustine compared to lomustine alone in recurrent glioblastoma [46]. A phase II study of VEGF Trap (aflibercept), a recombinantly produced fusion protein that captures circulating VEGF and CT-322, showed minimal evidence of single-agent activity in recurrent malignant glioma [47]. Other antiangiogenic agents evaluated include enzastaurin, an inhibitor of protein kinase C-beta that targets VEGF as well as the mTOR pathway [27]. The phase III trial of enzastaurin compared to lomustine in recurrent glioblastoma concluded that enzastaurin did not have superior efficacy compared to lomustine [27].

Similarly trials targeting epidermal growth factor receptor (EGFR) using agents such as erlotinib and gefitinib have shown limited activity in recurrent glioblastoma [48–51]. Irreversible EGFR inhibitors such as afatinib did not show efficacy when used in alone or combination with temozolomide in recurrent GBM [52]. There is an ongoing phase II study with second-generation EGFR inhibitor, dacomitinib (NCT01112527). Other targeted agents including the mammalian target of rapamycin (mTOR) inhibitor, temsirolimus, and the farnesyl transferase inhibitor, tipifarnib, have shown minimal activity in recurrent glioblastoma [53–57].

3.3.1 Summary and Recommendation

For recurrent glioblastoma, we recommend participation in a clinical trial. In case the patient is not eligible for a clinical trial and has good performance status, we suggest systemic therapy often with a non-bevacizumab regimen such as lomustine. We use bevacizumab-based regimens for patients with symptoms related to a significant component of vasogenic edema or patients who have significant steroid requirements or intolerance. For patients who need bevacizumab and have not received lomustine, we prefer the combination of bevacizumab with lomustine (Level II evidence) (Tables 1 and 2).

References

1. Stupp R, Mason WP, van den Bent MJ et al (2005) Radiotherapy plus concomitant and adjuvant temozolomide for glioblastoma. N Engl J Med 352:987–996
2. Stupp R, Hegi ME, Mason WP et al (2009) Effects of radiotherapy with concomitant and adjuvant temozolomide versus radiotherapy alone on survival in glioblastoma in a randomised phase III study: 5-year analysis of the EORTC-NCIC trial. Lancet Oncol 10:459–466
3. Hegi ME, Diserens AC, Gorlia T et al (2005) MGMT gene silencing and benefit from temozolomide in glioblastoma. N Engl J Med 352:997–1003
4. Clarke JL, Iwamoto FM, Sul J et al (2009) Randomized phase II trial of chemoradiotherapy followed by either dose-dense or metronomic temozolomide for newly diagnosed glioblastoma. J Clin Oncol 27:3861–3867
5. Gilbert MR, Wang M, Aldape KD et al (2013) Dose-dense temozolomide for newly diagnosed glioblastoma: a randomized phase III clinical trial. J Clin Oncol 31:4085–4091

6. Chalmers AJ (2009) The potential role and application of PARP inhibitors in cancer treatment. Br Med Bull 89:23–40
7. Dungey FA, Loser DA, Chalmers AJ (2008) Replication-dependent radiosensitization of human glioma cells by inhibition of poly(ADP-ribose) polymerase: mechanisms and therapeutic potential. Int J Radiat Oncol Biol Phys 72:1188–1197
8. Sandhu SK, Yap TA, de Bono JS (2010) Poly(ADP-ribose) polymerase inhibitors in cancer treatment: a clinical perspective. Eur J Cancer 46:9–20
9. Westphal M, Hilt DC, Bortey E et al (2003) A phase 3 trial of local chemotherapy with biodegradable carmustine (BCNU) wafers (Gliadel wafers) in patients with primary malignant glioma. Neuro-oncology 5:79–88
10. Duntze J, Litre CF, Eap C et al (2013) Implanted carmustine wafers followed by concomitant radiochemotherapy to treat newly diagnosed malignant gliomas: prospective, observational, multicenter study on 92 cases. Ann Surg Oncol 20:2065–2072
11. Folkman J (1971) Tumor angiogenesis: therapeutic implications. N Engl J Med 285:1182–1186
12. Carmeliet P, Jain RK (2011) Molecular mechanisms and clinical applications of angiogenesis. Nature 473:298–307
13. Ahluwalia MS, Gladson CL (2010) Progress on antiangiogenic therapy for patients with malignant glioma. J Oncol 2010:689018
14. Kleihues P, Louis DN, Scheithauer BW et al (2002) The WHO classification of tumors of the nervous system. J Neuropathol Exp Neurol 61:215–225
15. Wen PY, Kesari S (2008) Malignant gliomas in adults. N Engl J Med 359:492–507
16. Seidel S, Garvalov BK, Wirta V et al (2010) A hypoxic niche regulates glioblastoma stem cells through hypoxia inducible factor 2 alpha. Brain 133:983–995
17. Nam DH, Park K, Suh YL, Kim JH (2004) Expression of VEGF and brain specific angiogenesis inhibitor-1 in glioblastoma: prognostic significance. Oncol Rep 11:863–869
18. Robles Irizarry L, Hambardzumyan D, Nakano I, Gladson CL, Ahluwalia MS (2012) Therapeutic targeting of VEGF in the treatment of glioblastoma. Expert Opin Ther Targets 16:973–984
19. Gilbert MR, Dignam JJ, Armstrong TS et al (2014) A randomized trial of bevacizumab for newly diagnosed glioblastoma. N Engl J Med 370:699–708
20. Chinot OL, Wick W, Mason W et al (2014) Bevacizumab plus radiotherapy-temozolomide for newly diagnosed glioblastoma. N Engl J Med 370:709–722
21. Herrlinger U, Schaefer N, Steinbach JP et al (2013) Bevacizumab, irinotecan, and radiotherapy versus standard temozolomide and radiotherapy in newly diagnosed, MGMT-non-methylated glioblastoma patients: first results from the randomized multicenter GLARIUS trial. J Clin Oncol (Meeting Abstracts):31(18_suppl LBA2000)
22. Reardon DA, Fink KL, Mikkelsen T et al (2008) Randomized phase II study of cilengitide, an integrin-targeting arginine-glycine-aspartic acid peptide, in recurrent glioblastoma multiforme. J Clin Oncol 26:5610–5617
23. Stupp R, Hegi ME, Neyns B et al (2010) Phase I/IIa study of cilengitide and temozolomide with concomitant radiotherapy followed by cilengitide and temozolomide maintenance therapy in patients with newly diagnosed glioblastoma. J Clin Oncol 28:2712–2718
24. Stupp R, Hegi ME, Gorlia T et al (2013) Cilengitide combined with standard treatment for patients with newly diagnosed glioblastoma and methylated O6-methylguanine-DNA methyltransferase (MGMT) gene promoter: key results of the multicenter, randomized, open-label, controlled, phase III CENTRIC study. J Clin Oncol (Meeting Abstracts):31 (18_suppl LBA2009)
25. Nabors LB, Fink KL, Mikkelsen T et al (2013) Randomized phase II study investigating cilengitide added to standard chemoradiotherapy in patients with newly diagnosed glioblastoma with unmethylated 06-methylguanine-DNA methyltransferase (MGMT) gene promoter: initial report of the CORE study. In: European cancer congress, Amsterdam
26. Brandes AA, Tosoni A, Amista P et al (2004) How effective is BCNU in recurrent glioblastoma in the modern era? a phase II trial. Neurology 63:1281–1284

27. Wick W, Puduvalli VK, Chamberlain MC et al (2010) Phase III study of enzastaurin compared with lomustine in the treatment of recurrent intracranial glioblastoma. J Clin Oncol 28:1168–1174
28. Field KM, Simes J, Wheeler H et al (2013) A randomized phase II study of carboplatin and bevacizumab in recurrent glioblastoma multiforme (CABARET). J Clin Oncol (Meeting Abstracts):31(15_suppl 2017)
29. Schmidt F, Fischer J, Herrlinger U, Dietz K, Dichgans J, Weller M (2006) PCV chemotherapy for recurrent glioblastoma. Neurology 66:587–589
30. Wick A, Felsberg J, Steinbach JP et al (2007) Efficacy and tolerability of temozolomide in an alternating weekly regimen in patients with recurrent glioma. J Clin Oncol 25:3357–3361
31. Norden AD, Lesser GJ, Drappatz J et al (2013) Phase 2 study of dose-intense temozolomide in recurrent glioblastoma. Neuro Oncol 15:930–935
32. Perry JR, Belanger K, Mason WP et al (2010) Phase II trial of continuous dose-intense temozolomide in recurrent malignant glioma: RESCUE study. J Clin Oncol 28:2051–2057
33. Omuro A, Chan TA, Abrey LE et al (2013) Phase II trial of continuous low-dose temozolomide for patients with recurrent malignant glioma. Neuro Oncol 15:242–250
34. Brem H, Piantadosi S, Burger PC et al (1995) Placebo-controlled trial of safety and efficacy of intraoperative controlled delivery by biodegradable polymers of chemotherapy for recurrent gliomas. The polymer-brain tumor treatment group. Lancet 345:1008–1012
35. Stark-Vance V (2005) Bevacizumab and CPT-11 in the treatment of relapsed malignant glioma. Neuro Oncol 7:369
36. Vredenburgh JJ, Desjardins A, Herndon JE 2nd et al (2007) Bevacizumab plus irinotecan in recurrent glioblastoma multiforme. J Clin Oncol 25:4722–4729
37. Friedman HS, Prados MD, Wen PY et al (2009) Bevacizumab alone and in combination with irinotecan in recurrent glioblastoma. J Clin Oncol 27:4733–4740
38. Kreisl TN, Kim L, Moore K et al (2009) Phase II trial of single-agent bevacizumab followed by bevacizumab plus irinotecan at tumor progression in recurrent glioblastoma. J Clin Oncol 27:740–745
39. Reardon DA, Desjardins A, Vredenburgh JJ et al (2009) Metronomic chemotherapy with daily, oral etoposide plus bevacizumab for recurrent malignant glioma: a phase II study. Br J Cancer 101:1986–1994
40. Reardon DA, Desjardins A, Peters KB et al (2012) Phase II study of carboplatin, irinotecan, and bevacizumab for bevacizumab naive, recurrent glioblastoma. J Neurooncol 107:155–164
41. Desjardins A, Reardon DA, Coan A et al (2012) Bevacizumab and daily temozolomide for recurrent glioblastoma. Cancer 118:1302–1312
42. Raizer JJ, Grimm S, Chamberlain MC et al (2010) A phase 2 trial of single-agent bevacizumab given in an every-3-week schedule for patients with recurrent high-grade gliomas. Cancer 116:5297–5305
43. Bokstein F, Shpigel S, Blumenthal DT (2008) Treatment with bevacizumab and irinotecan for recurrent high-grade glial tumors. Cancer 112:2267–2273
44. Taal W, Oosterkamp HM, Walenkamp AME et al (2013) A randomized phase II study of bevacizumab versus bevacizumab plus lomustine versus lomustine single agent in recurrent glioblastoma: the Dutch BELOB study. J Clin Oncol (Meeting Abstracts):31(15_suppl 2001)
45. Batchelor TT, Sorensen AG, di Tomaso E et al (2007) AZD2171, a pan-VEGF receptor tyrosine kinase inhibitor, normalizes tumor vasculature and alleviates edema in glioblastoma patients. Cancer Cell 11:83–95
46. Batchelor TT, Mulholland P, Neyns B et al (2013) Phase III randomized trial comparing the efficacy of cediranib as monotherapy, and in combination with lomustine, versus lomustine alone in patients with recurrent glioblastoma. J Clin Oncol 31:3212–3218
47. de Groot JF, Lamborn KR, Chang SM et al (2011) Phase II study of aflibercept in recurrent malignant glioma: a North American brain tumor consortium study. J Clin Oncol 29:2689–2695
48. Prados MD, Yung WK, Jaeckle KA et al (2004) Phase 1 trial of irinotecan (CPT-11) in patients with recurrent malignant glioma: a North American brain tumor consortium study. Neuro Oncol 6:44–54

49. Krishnan S, Brown PD, Ballman KV et al (2006) Phase I trial of erlotinib with radiation therapy in patients with glioblastoma multiforme: results of North central cancer treatment group protocol N0177. Int J Radiat Oncol Biol Phys 65:1192–1199
50. Rich JN, Reardon DA, Peery T et al (2004) Phase II trial of gefitinib in recurrent glioblastoma. J Clin Oncol 22:133–142
51. van den Bent MJ, Brandes AA, Rampling R et al (2009) Randomized phase II trial of erlotinib versus temozolomide or carmustine in recurrent glioblastoma: EORTC brain tumor group study 26034. J Clin Oncol 27:1268–1274
52. Eisenstat DD, Nabors LB, Mason WP et al (2011) A phase II study of daily afatinib (BIBW 2992) with or without temozolomide (21/28 days) in the treatment of patients with recurrent glioblastoma. J Clin Oncol (Meeting Abstracts):29(15_suppl 2010)
53. Chang SM, Wen P, Cloughesy T et al (2005) Phase II study of CCI-779 in patients with recurrent glioblastoma multiforme. Invest New Drugs 23:357–361
54. Cloughesy TF, Wen PY, Robins HI et al (2006) Phase II trial of tipifarnib in patients with recurrent malignant glioma either receiving or not receiving enzyme-inducing antiepileptic drugs: a North American brain tumor consortium study. J Clin Oncol 24:3651–3656
55. Doherty L, Gigas DC, Kesari S et al (2006) Pilot study of the combination of EGFR and mTOR inhibitors in recurrent malignant gliomas. Neurology 67:156–158
56. Galanis E, Buckner JC, Maurer MJ et al (2005) Phase II trial of temsirolimus (CCI-779) in recurrent glioblastoma multiforme: a North central cancer treatment group study. J Clin Oncol 23:5294–5304
57. Reardon DA, Desjardins A, Vredenburgh JJ et al (2010) Phase 2 trial of erlotinib plus sirolimus in adults with recurrent glioblastoma. J Neurooncol 96:219–230

Novel Chemotherapeutic Approaches in Adult High-Grade Gliomas

Justin T. Jordan and Patrick Y. Wen

Abstract Despite decades of advancing science and clinical trials, average survival remains dismal for individuals with high-grade gliomas. Our understanding of the genetic and molecular aberrations that contribute to the aggressive nature of these tumors is continually growing, as is our ability to target such specific traits. Herein, we review the major classes of such targeted therapies, as well as the relevant clinical trial outcomes regarding their efficacy.

Keywords Glioma · Glioblastoma · Targeted therapy · Chemotherapy

Contents

J.T. Jordan · P.Y. Wen (✉)
Center for Neuro-Oncology, Dana-Farber/Brigham and Women's Cancer Center, 450 Brookline Avenue, Boston, MA 02215, USA
e-mail: pwen@partners.org

P.Y. Wen
Division of Neuro-Oncology, Department of Neurology, Brigham and Women's Hospital, Harvard Medical School, 75 Francis Street, Boston, MA 02115, USA

J. Raizer and A. Parsa (eds.), *Current Understanding and Treatment of Gliomas*, Cancer Treatment and Research 163, DOI 10.1007/978-3-319-12048-5_8

1 Introduction

Despite decades of advancing science and clinical trials, survival remains dismal for individuals with high-grade gliomas [1]. In 2005, in the setting of ill-defined treatment strategies with radiation and alkylating chemotherapy agents, the landmark publication by Stupp and colleagues changed the standard of care for patients with glioblastoma. Using concurrent radiation and temozolomide, followed by adjuvant temozolomide, patients' overall survival improved from 12.1 to 14.6 months over radiation alone [2]. Further, two-year survival improved from 10.4 % to 26.5 % [2]. This study represents the greatest advancement in modern neuro-oncology therapy, but still leaves ample room for improvement.

In the years since Stupp's publication, overall survival numbers have improved marginally in various centers, though the next great breakthrough in high-grade glioma care is still on the horizon. Whereas temozolomide remains the backbone of chemotherapy for these tumors, and other alkylating agents such as lomustine in the recurrent setting, alternative and targeted chemotherapy approaches remain actively under investigation. The following is a summary of the major classes of such novel chemotherapy strategies that have been studied in clinical trials (Fig. 1).

2 Vascular Endothelial Growth Factor

Vascular neogenesis is a pathologic hallmark of glioblastoma, and has been a major focus of study in neuro-oncology for decades (Tables 1, 2). Angiogenesis is controlled through a complex network of pro- and antiangiogenic blood vessels, and chief among these is vascular endothelial growth factor (VEGF) and its receptor, vascular endothelial growth factor receptor (VEGFR).

Capitalizing on this translational knowledge, bevacizumab, a recombinant humanized monoclonal antibody against VEGF-A, came into the landscape as one of the first antiangiogenic agents. Based on reported successes in other systemic cancers, two early phase II studies for recurrent glioblastoma used bevacizumab and irinotecan (a topoisomerase I inhibitor) and demonstrated 60 % radiographic response and a 6-month progression-free survival (PFS) of 38–46 % [3, 4]. The larger randomized phase II BRAIN trial was later performed, evaluating the activity of bevacizumab with or without iriniotecan in recurrent glioblastoma, and showed radiographic response in 38 and 28 %, respectively, and 6-month PFS was 50 and 42 %, respectively [5]. Around the same time, a single-arm phase II study of

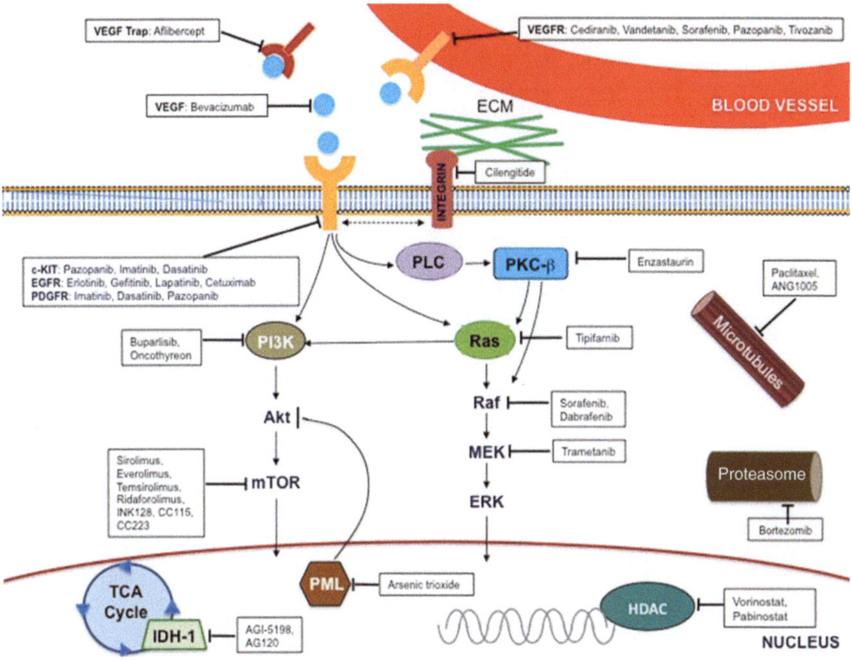

Fig. 1 Schematic representing select targeted therapies for which clinical trial results are available in high-grade gliomas. Edited with permission from Lee et al. "current and future directions for Phase II trials in high-grade glioma." Expert reviews in Neurotherapeutics. 13(4), 369–387 (2013). ECM: Extracellular matrix, EGFR: Epithelial growth factor receptor, HDAC: Histone deacetylase, IDH1: Isocitrate dehydrogenase-1, PDGFR: Platelet-derived growth factor receptor, PML: Promyelocytic leukemia, VEGFR: Vascular endothelial growth factor receptor

bevacizumab alone was published for recurrent glioblastoma and showed radiographic response in 35 % of patients, and a 29 % 6-month PFS [6]. Based on these studies, the FDA granted accelerated approval of bevacizumab for recurrent glioblastoma, contingent upon subsequent phase III study [7].

In response to this requirement by the FDA, two large phase III, randomized trials were subsequently published in newly diagnosed glioblastoma. The AVAglio trial, an international, industry-sponsored, randomized trial, evaluated bevacizumab versus placebo in addition to standard chemoradiation with temozolomide [8]. With co-primary endpoints of PFS and overall survival (OS), the predefined PFS significance level was met (10.6 vs. 6.2 months), though the target OS significance endpoint was not met (16.8 vs. 16.7 months) [8]. Simultaneously published, the RTOG 0825 study was also as a phase III, randomized trial in newly diagnosed glioblastoma patients. Similar to AVAglio, this was designed to compare bevacizumab versus placebo in combination with standard chemoradiation with temozolomide, with a planned crossover [9]. With co-primary endpoints of PFS and OS, the bevacizumab arm did not meet either predetermined PFS (10.7 vs. 7.3 months) or

Table 1 Selected antiangiogenic therapy trials in recurrent high-grade gliomas

Drug	Target	Combinations	Phase	PFS (week)	OS (week)	References
Bevacizumab	VEGF Ab	Alone	II	16	31	Kreisl [6]
		Irinotecan	II	20–24	31–42	Vrendenburgh [3, 4], Friedman [5], Moller [11]
		Irinotecan + cetuximab	II	16	29	Hasselbalch [12]
		Carboplatin	II	23	33	Reardon [13]
		Sorafenib	II	21	36	Galanis [14]
		Temozolomide	II	16	37	Desjardins [15]
		Erlotinib	II	18	45	Sathornsumetee [16]
		Temsirolimus	II	8	15	Lassen [17]
		Etoposide	II	18	46	Reardon [18]
		Fotemustine	II	21	36	Soffietti [19]
Aflibercept	VEGF Trap	Alone	II	12–24	39–55	De Groot [21]
Cediranib	VEGFR TKI	Alone	II	17	32	Batchelor [23]
		Alone, versus lomustine, or + lomustine	III	13 versus 12 versus 18	32 versus 39 versus 38	Batchelor [24]
Vandetanib	VEGFR EGFR TKI	Alone	I/II	5–7	19–30	Kreisl [26]

(continued)

Table 1 (continued)

Drug	Target	Combinations	Phase	PFS (week)	OS (week)	References
Sorafenib	VEGFR PDGFR RAF TKI	Temozolomide	II	6–13	30–41	Reardon [27] Zustovich [28]
		Bevacizumab	II	12	22	Galanis [14]
		Erlotinib	II	10	22	Peereboom [29]
		Temsirolimus	I/II	8	NR	Lee [31]
Pazopanib	VEGFR PDGFR c-KIT	Alone	II	12	35	Iwamoto [32]
		Lapatinib	II	8	NR	Reardon [33]
Enzastaurin	PKC-β	Alone	I	22	51	Rampling [34]
		Alone, vs Lomustine	III	6 versus 6	NR, NR	Wick [35]
Cilengitide	Integrins αvβ3 αvβ5	Alone	I	NR	22	Nabors [40]
		Alone	II	8	39	Reardon [41] Gilbert [42]

EGFR Epithelial growth factor receptor, *NR* Not reported, *PDGFR* Platelet-derived growth factor receptor, *RAF* Rapidly activated fibrosarcoma, *TKI* Tyrosine kinase inhibitor, *VEGF* Vascular endothelial growth factor, *VEGFR* Vascular endothelial growth factor receptor

Table 2 Selected antiangiogenic therapy trials in newly diagnosed high-grade gliomas (Gilbert [9])

Drug	Target	Combinations	Phase	PFS (week)	OS (month)	References
Bevacizumab	VEGF	RT + TMZ	III	42	62–67	Chinot [8]
Sorafenib	VEGFR PDGFR RAF TKI	RT + TMZ	II	24	52	Hainsworth [30]
Cilengitide	Integrins αvβ3 αvβ5	RT + TMZ	I/IIa	32	64	Stupp [44]
		RT + TMZ	II	40	79	Nabors [43]
		RT + TMZ	III	24	69	Nabors [46]
		RT + TMZ	III	58	113	Stupp [45]

VEGF Vascular endothelial growth factor, *VEGFR* Vascular endothelial growth factor receptor, *PDGFR* Platelet-derived growth factor receptor

OS (15.7 vs. 16.1 months) levels of significance. The studies also evaluated quality of life measures and durability of functional status, and AVAglio found benefit from bevacizumab whereas RTOG 0825 found detriment by the addition of bevacizumab. Following these mixed results, it is unclear whether the FDA will grant full approval of bevacizumab and the field anxiously awaits further developments.

Aside from FDA-required study, many additional phase II bevacizumab-based combination trials have been performed for recurrent glioblastoma [10]. Bevacizumab with irinotecan has been reported by several groups, with PFS ranging from 20 to 24 weeks, and OS from 31 to 42 weeks [3–5, 11]. Bevacizumab and irinotecan combined with cetuximab (an EGFR inhibitor, see below) was reported with a PFS of 16 weeks and an OS of 29 weeks [12], and combined with carboplatin had a PFS of 23 weeks and an OS of 33 weeks was reported [13]. Combinations of bevacizumab and sorafenib (a multi-targeted tyrosine kinase inhibitor, see below) had a PFS of 21 weeks and an OS of 36 weeks [14], bevacizumab and temozolomide had a PFS of 16 weeks and an OS of 37 weeks [15], bevacizumab and erlotinib (an epidermal growth factor (EGFR) inhibitor, see below) had 18 weeks PFS and 45 week OS [16], and bevacizumab and temsirolimus (an mTOR inhibitor, see below) had 8 week PFS and 15 week OS [17]. Finally, employing older chemotherapy drugs, studies of bevacizumab with etoposide had a PFS of 18 weeks and an OS of 46 weeks [18], and with fotemustine had a PFS of 21 weeks and an OS of 36 weeks [19]. Although these prospective studies are not easily compared due to their small size, varying regimens and patient populations, the general consensus has been that no combination reported to date surpasses outcomes of bevacizumab monotherapy for recurrent high-grade gliomas [20].

Aside from bevacizumab, another means of removing the angiogenic effect of VEGF is to remove the ligand itself. Aflibercept is a fusion protein that scavenges both VEGF and placental growth factor from patients, inhibiting angiogenesis. One trial of aflibercept has been published in adults with recurrent high-grade gliomas and showed moderate toxicity but minimal activity with a PFS of 24 weeks for patients with anaplastic tumors and only 12 weeks for patients with glioblastoma, suggesting limited utility as a monotherapy in these patients [21]. Further study has, therefore, not been sought.

3 Integrins

Integrins regulate cell adhesion and are important in tumor growth, invasion, and angiogenesis [22, 23]. Cilengitide is a selective integrin inhibitor, targeting $\alpha v\beta 3$ and $\alpha v\beta 5$ integrins, and has been studied in multiple trials for recurrent gliomas. A phase I study of cilengitide monotherapy for recurrent high-grade gliomas demonstrated adequate drug tolerability and safety, with sustained tumor responses that correlated with decreased MRI perfusion [24]. A phase II trial in recurrent glioblastoma showed modest antitumor results, with an overall survival of 9.9 months and 6-month progression-free survival of 15 %, trending better with higher doses of medication [25]. In a surgical trial, designed to prove drug delivery to recurrent glioblastoma, patients received cilengitide for 3 doses before tumor resection, then continued for up to 2 years after surgery [26]. Cilengitide was detected in all tumors, demonstrating adequate delivery, but led to a 6-month progression-free survival of only 12 % [26]. From this, the authors suggested that combination studies with cilengitide might be more efficacious.

Further, several newly diagnosed glioblastoma trials have been performed with cilengitide. In a phase II dose-randomized trial of cilengitide plus temozolomide and radiation in newly diagnosed glioblastoma, comparing to historical controls, adequate tolerability was found with an average overall survival of 19.7 months, which was better than 14.6 months in their historical control [27]. Notably, this benefit was seen regardless of MGMT methylation status. Another single-arm phase I/II study of cilengitide with concurrent radiation and temozolomide, followed by adjuvant cilengitide and temozolomide demonstrated good tolerability with an overall survival benefit in those patients with MGMT promoter methylation [28]. The follow-up phase III CENTRIC study, however, demonstrated no statistical benefit of adding cilengitide to standard chemoradiation for MGMT-methylated patients, with PFS of 10.7 months for control and 13.5 months for cilengitide, and 26.3 month OS in both arms [29]. For newly diagnosed glioblastoma patients without MGMT methylation, the phase II CORE study showed a modest survival advantage in adding cilengitide to standard radiation and temozolomide, with PFS of 4.1 months for control, 5.6 months for twice weekly cilengitide, and 5.9 months for five times weekly cilengitide during radiation, then twice weekly cilengitide thereafter [30]. These poor results ended the development of cilengitide for treatment of high-grade gliomas.

4 Tyrosine Kinase Inhibitors

Among the largest and most promising classes of antineoplastic agents are tyrosine kinase inhibitors (TKI) which target receptor tyrosine kinases (RTKs), the phosphorylating enzymes that control signaling cascades for cell growth and survival. The most commonly upregulated or activated RTKs in glioblastoma include epithelial growth factor receptor (EGFR), VEGFR, and platelet-derived growth factor receptor (PDGFR). Downstream, two of the most constitutively activated pathways in glioblastoma signal through rat sarcoma (RAS) and phosphatidylinositol 3-kinase (PI3K), which have activating mutations in up to 88 % of cases [31]. Further, mutations in inhibitory signaling proteins, such as phosphatase and tensin homolog (PTEN) and neurofibromatosis 1 (NF1), are commonly seen in glioblastoma and promote RTK signaling activation and cell survival [31]. By pharmacologically inhibiting particular RTKs in the aforementioned signaling cascades, downstream proteins and cell functions may also be inhibited. Many such therapeutics have been studied and are summarized below (Table 3).

The small molecule inhibitors that make up TKIs are generally orally bioavailable, but many have poor penetration across the blood–brain barrier (BBB) or are substrates of drug efflux pumps. Additional difficulties with the class include off target effects, leading to unwanted side effects, as well as drug resistance due to upregulation of parallel signaling cascades (Table 3).

5 Vascular Endothelial Growth Factor Receptor

With the advantage of oral bioavailability, a large number of VEGFR-targeting TKIs have been examined in patients with glioblastomas. The hope has been for a robust antiangiogenic effect, translating into targeted antitumor efficacy, and improving upon the success of bevacizumab.

Cediranib, a potent VEGFR-targeting TKI, is the most extensively studied of these. A phase II clinical trial of cediranib alone for recurrent glioblastoma was initially encouraging, showing a 6-month PFS of 26 %, and radiographic response in 57 % of patients when measured as >50 % reduction in contrast enhancing volume [32]. However, in employing the Macdonald criteria, only 27 % radiographic response was seen [32]. A phase III trial of cediranib monotherapy versus cediranib and lomustine versus lomustine monotherapy showed that the addition of cediranib to lomustine provided no benefit [33]. Further study of cediranib using MRI perfusion showed that only a small subset of patients receiving this drug demonstrated a decrease in perfusion, which was ultimately associated with better clinical responses [34]. This implies that some patients may respond well to cediranib, but identifying those individuals up-front remains a challenge.

Table 3 Selected clinical trials of tyrosine kinase inhibitors in high-grade gliomas

Drug	Target	Combinations	Disease stage	Phase	PFS (wk)	OS (wk)	References
Erlotinib	EGFR	Alone versus TMZ or BCNU	Recurrent	II	7 versus 10	32 versus 31	van den Bent [50]
		Bev versus Bev alone	Recurrent	II	42 versus 22	72 versus 28	D'Alessandris [51]
		Bevacizumab	Recurrent	II	18	45	Sathornsumetee [16]
		Temsirolimus	Recurrent	I/II	8	NR	Wen [52]
		Sirolimus	Recurrent	I	4	NR	Nghiemphu [53]
		Dasatinib	Recurrent	I	4	NR	Reardon [54]
		Sorafenib	Recurrent	II	10	23	Peereboom [29]
		RT + TMZ	Up-front	II	33	81	Prados [55]
		RT + TMZ	Up-front	I/II	29	65	Brown [56]
Gefitinib		Alone	Recurrent	II	8	39	Rich [61]
		Everolimus	Recurrent	I	10	24	Kreisl [62]
Lapatinib		Temozolomide	Recurrent	I	10	24	Karavasilis [65]
Imatinib	PDGFR	Alone	Up-front	II	NR	27	Razis [71]
		Alone	Recurrent	II	7	24	Raymond [72]
		Hydroxyurea	Recurrent	II	14	49	Reardon [76]
		Hydroxyurea	Recurrent	II	11	33	Desjardins [75]
		Hydroxyurea	Recurrent	II	6	26	Reardon [73]
Dasatinib		CCNU	Recurrent	I/II	5	28	Franceschi [77]
		Alone	Recurrent	II	7	32	Lassman [78]
Everolimus	mTOR	Neoadjuvant RT + TMZ, then + BEV	Up-front	II	49	60	Hainsworth [88]

(continued)

Table 3 (continued)

Drug	Target	Combinations	Disease stage	Phase	PFS (wk)	OS (wk)	References
Temsirolimus		Alone	Recurrent	II	9	19	Galanis [89]
		Bevacizumab	Recurrent	II	8	15	Lassen [17]
		Sorafenib	Recurrent	I/II	8	NR	Lee [31]
Tipifarnib	RAS	RT	Up-front	I	NR	52	Moyal [94]
		Before RT	Up-front	II	6	33	Lustig [95]

BEV Bevacizumab, *EGFR* Endothelial growth factor receptor, *mTOR* Mammalian target of rapamycin, *NR* Not reported, *PDGFR* Platelet-derived growth factor receptor, *RAS* Rat sarcoma, *RT* Radiation therapy, *TMZ* Temozolomide

Vandetanib is a multi-targeted TKI, which mainly affects VEGFR-2, as well as EGFR. This drug has been evaluated in one small phase I/II trial of recurrent high-grade gliomas and showed a 6-month PFS of 6.5 % in glioblastomas and 7 % in anaplastic gliomas, with overall survival of 6.3 months and 7.6 months, respectively [35]. Combinations of vandetanib with sirolimus and cilengitide have also failed to show any significant activity.

Sorafenib, another TKI-targeting VEGFR, as well as PDGFR and rapidly activated fibrosarcoma (RAF), has been investigated in several prospective trials. In two phase II studies of sorafenib and temozolomide for recurrent glioblastoma, 6-month PFS ranged from 9 to 26 %, with tolerable side effects, but less than robust antitumor effect [36, 37]. Similarly, when combining sorafenib with bevacizumab in recurrent glioblastoma, there was no survival advantage above historical controls of bevacizumab alone [14]. Finally, for recurrent glioblastoma, a phase II study of sorafenib and erlotinib (EGFR TKI, see below) did not meet its primary objective of 30 % increase in OS compared with historical controls [38]. In newly diagnosed glioblastoma, adding sorafenib to temozolomide after standard chemoradiation did not appear to improve efficacy of treatment compared to standard therapy [39]. Finally, a phase I/II trial combining sorafenib and temsirolimus (mTOR TKI, see below) for recurrent glioblastoma was terminated after the stage I portion due to lack of activity [40].

Pazopanib, another multi-targeted TKI, inhibits VEGFR, PDGFR, and c-KIT. A phase II study of pazopanib monotherapy in 35 recurrent glioblastoma patients was reasonably well tolerated, but did not prolong progression-free survival despite a moderate amount of radiographic response [41]. Also, a phase II evaluation of pazopanib and lapatinib (EGFR TKI, see below) was unsuccessful due to excessive dose-limiting toxicity and lack of efficacy [42].

Tivozanib is another VEGFR-targeting TKI, currently under investigation with no reported outcomes to date (ClinicalTrials.gov NCT01846871).

Downstream of VEGFR, β-protein kinase C (PKC-β) is involved in both PI3K and RAS pathways, and is inhibited by enzastaurin. One small phase I study of enzastaurin in recurrent glioblastoma reported a 5.5-month PFS and an 11.7-month OS [43]. Further, a phase III open-label study comparing enzastaurin versus lomustine for recurrent glioblastomas was terminated at interim analysis for futility, with a PFS of 1.5 versus 1.6 months and objective response in 2.9 % versus 4.3 %, respectively [44].

Following disease progression on a VEGFR-targeting TKI, one small study showed that using bevacizumab may still have efficacy after relapse. This implies that, although the biology of tumors may change after exposure to a VEGFR TKI, subsequent response to bevacizumab may not be ruled out [45, 46].

6 Epithelial Growth Factor Receptor

Approximately 40–90 % of glioblastomas overexpress epithelial growth factor receptor (EGFR), and 40–50 % are associated with high-level amplification of the EGFR gene [22, 47–49]. The relationship of this amplification to downstream mitogenic pathways, including RAS and PI3K/AKT cascades, makes it a potentially good therapeutic target. Further, approximately 40 % of GBM with EGFR amplifications also have EGFR mutations, especially EGFRvIII [22]. EGFR-targeted therapies in other cancers such as lung cancer have been clinically effective, so EGFR TKIs have been an area of active investigation in glioblastoma in recent years as well.

Erlotinib, the first of these EGFR TKIs, has been examined in several trials. A phase II trial comparing erlotinib monotherapy to either temozolomide or carmustine in recurrent glioblastoma was negative, as control arms did significantly better than erlotinib, with 6-month PFS of 24 % versus 11.4 %, respectively [50]. Also in recurrent high-grade gliomas, combining erlotinib and bevacizumab has shown mixed results, with positive findings in small, molecularly targeted patient population (PTEN retained, VEGF amplified, EGFRvIII positive) [51], but negative results in larger, more generalized patient populations [16]. Although combination of EGFR inhibitors with other complementary targeted agents may theoretically be more effective, these combinations have overall been poorly tolerated. In a phase I/II study erlotinib and temsirolimus (mTOR TKI, see below) in recurrent high-grade glioma patients, significant toxicity was encountered and the maximum tolerated dose of temsirolimus in this combination was less than 10 % of the single-agent effective dose and no activity was observed with a 6-month PFS of only 13 % [52]. Another phase I study evaluating the combination of erlotinib and sirolimus (mTOR TKI, see below) for recurrent malignant gliomas similarly found significant toxicity with minimal effect on PFS [53]. Phase I study of combined erlotinib and dasatinib (PDGFR TKI, see below) in recurrent glioblastoma identified safe doses of both, but showed no radiographic response and only a 2 % 6-month PFS [54]. Finally, a phase II study of erlotinib and sorafenib in recurrent glioblastoma did not meet its primary objective of 30 % increase in OS compared with historical controls [29]. In two newly diagnosed glioblastoma trials, using erlotinib in addition to standard temozolomide and radiation showed improvement of OS from 14.1 months historical control to 19.3 months in one study [55], but no significant benefit over historical control in the other [56].

Given the high frequency of EGFR amplification and mutations in glioblastomas, several authors have attempted to stratify erlotinib outcomes by amplification status, with a positive correlation in one study [57], but no such correlation in others [50, 58]. Additionally, patients expressing the variant receptor EGFRvIII showed stronger responses to erlotinib in early study when PTEN wild type was also present [59], though this correlation has not been reproducible in other studies [50, 56, 60].

Gefitinib, another EGFR TKI, has been studied in multiple trials of high-grade glioma. In recurrent glioblastoma, gefitinib monotherapy showed a disappointing

6-month PFS of 13 % [61]. A phase I study of gefitinib and everolimus (mTOR inhibitor, see below) in recurrent glioblastoma also found minimal response, with only one of 22 patients progression free at six months [62]. Similar to erlotinib, EGFR expression levels apparently did not correlate with responsiveness to this drug [61], nor did EGFR mutational status [63].

The final EGFR TKI studied in high-grade gliomas is lapatinib, which also inhibits erbB2. A phase I/II study of lapatinib monotherapy for recurrent glioblastoma was stopped early due to lack of clinical effect, and did not show clinical correlation with EGFRvIII expression or PTEN loss [64]. Later, a phase I study of lapatinib and temozolomide in recurrent high-grade gliomas showed moderate toxicity with still limited effect on PFS and OS, at 2.4 and 5.9 months respectively [65]. Again, the authors looked at EGFR amplification and EGFRvIII expression and found no correlation with PFS [65]. A phase I/II evaluation of lapatinib and pazopanib was negative. Although it did not reach the maximum-tolerated doses in phase I, phase II pharmacokinetic studies indicated a level of lapatinib that was subtherapeutic for target blockade [33]. In a proof-of-concept study, after one week of standard dose lapatinib for recurrent glioblastoma, surgically resected tissue demonstrated lapatinib sequestration with concentrations greater than the IC50 in xenograft models, though still below the concentration reported as necessary to induce cell death in cell lines. Further, evaluation of EGFR phosphorylation levels in preoperatively treated tumors demonstrated suboptimal target effect by the intratumoral concentrations achieved [66]. Notably, there are data to suggest that first generation EGFR-targeting TKIs are best efficacious against EGFR kinase domain mutations as is seen in lung cancers, whereas lapatinib targets EGFR extracellular domain mutations which are more common in glioblastoma [66]. However, lapatinib does not achieve adequate concentrations with standard daily dosing, and so weekly pulse dosing of lapatinib is being examined for greater tissue delivery.

Overall, monotherapy with EGFR TKIs has been disappointing, primarily because of the poor penetration of the available agents across the BBB. Studies evaluating pulse dosing to achieve higher C_{max} in genetically enriched populations, or newer agents with improved penetration across the BBB such as dacomitinib which is under study now (ClinicalTrials.gov NCT01112527, NCT01520870), may potentially be more beneficial.

7 Platelet-Derived Growth Factor Receptor

Another important receptor tyrosine kinase in tumor growth and survival is PDGFR, which is amplified or mutated in approximately 10 % of glioblastomas [67]. Tyrosine kinase inhibitors targeting PDGFR include imatinib and dasatinib, which will be reviewed here, as well as pazopanib, which even more strongly targets VEGFR and is included in that section (above).

Imatinib, targeting PDGFR as well as several other RTKs (including ABL and KIT), has been successfully used in several cancers including chronic myeloid lymphoma and gastrointestinal stromal cell tumors [68, 69]. In trials for both newly diagnosed [70] and recurrent GBM [71–73], imatinib has been well tolerated but had minimal activity alone or in combination with hydroxyurea [74, 75]. The lack of efficacy may be related to the fact that imatinib is a P-glycoprotein substrate and has poor penetration across the BBB.

Dasatinib, targeting PDGFR as well as c-KIT, ABL, and Scr family kinases, has also been investigated in recurrent malignant gliomas. A study of dasatinib and lomustine for recurrent glioblastoma found significant hematologic side effects leading to suboptimal tolerance among patients, with a PFS of only 1.3 months [76]. A phase II study of dasatinib monotherapy conducted by the Radiation Therapy Oncology Group (RTOG 0627) also failed to show any significant benefit [77]. Finally, a retrospective study evaluated the addition of dasatinib to bevacizumab in patients with recurrent glioblastomas who failed bevacizumab therapy, and found no significant benefit [78]. The Alliance for Clinical Trials in Oncology is currently evaluating the combination of dasatinib with standard chemoradiation in newly diagnosed glioblastoma (ClinicalTrials.gov NCT00869401) and with bevacizumab in recurrent glioblastomas (ClinicalTrials.gov NCT00892177).

8 PI3K/AKT/mTOR

Phosphatidylinositol 3-kinase (PI3K) signaling is activated in the majority of glioblastoma patients, either as a result of mutations in PI3K subunit genes PIK3Ca or PIK3R1 (15–20 %) or through loss of the tumor suppressor gene *Phosphatase and Tensin Homolog* (PTEN) (40 %) or through activation of receptor tyrosine kinases such as EGFR (45 %) [22, 79]. This signaling cascade is important for cell growth, proliferation, and survival. The downstream effectors of PI3K include AKT and mammalian target of rapamycin (mTOR) which, through mTOR complex (mTORC)-1 and -2, plays key roles in cell metabolism, survival, cytoskeletal production, and protein translation. PI3K activation is associated with poor prognosis in glioblastoma [80].

Among PI3K-targeting drugs, one of the most thoroughly studied is buparlisib, a pan-PI3K inhibitor. In a phase I study of buparlisib monotherapy for recurrent advanced solid tumors, the drug was well tolerated and demonstrated antitumor activity [81]. It is notable that among the more common adverse events reported in this trial, buparlisib was associated with mood disturbance, a new TKI-related side effect [81]. A phase II study of buparlisib in recurrent glioblastoma patients demonstrated adequate tumor concentrations to inhibit the PI3K pathway (as evidenced by reduction of phosphorylated AKT), though there were no data to suggest single-agent efficacy [82]. Ongoing studies with buparlisib include a phase I dose-escalation trial with concurrent standard chemoradiation in newly diagnosed glioblastoma (ClinicalTrials.gov NCT01473901), and combination trials for recurrent glioblastoma with bevacizumab (ClinicalTrials.gov NCT01349660), and carboplatin or lomustine (ClinicalTrials.gov NCT01934361).

Another PI3K inhibitor under study is PX-866 (oncothyreon), a semisynthetic derivative of wortmannin which irreversibly inhibits PI3K. A phase I study of PX-866 for advanced solid tumors showed that the drug was well tolerated and 22 % of patients obtained stable disease [83]. There is an ongoing single-agent phase II study of PX-866 in recurrent glioblastoma (ClinicalTrials.gov NCT01259869).

Also in the PI3K pathway, mTOR has been a major focus of trials given both the importance of mTOR for mitogenesis, as well as the dual pathway activation of mTOR by way of either RAS or PI3K. Rapamycin (sirolimus), the drug for which mTOR is named, has received little clinical study in glioblastoma. In one proof-of-concept phase I trial in PTEN-deficient glioblastomas using presurgical dosing of rapamycin, intratumoral rapamycin concentrations were sufficient in all patients, though inhibitory effect on mTOR was variable [84]. Markers of tumor cell proliferation were reduced in half of patients after one week of rapamycin, though in as many patients AKT activation was seen due to lack of negative feedback, and time to progression was significantly less [84].

Everolimus, another mTOR inhibitor, has been studied in multiple trials. A phase I study of everolimus and temozolomide in combination with radiation therapy in newly diagnosed glioblastoma showed acceptable tolerance, and imaging with FDG-PET showed decreased tumor metabolic activity in a subset of patients [85]. A second, similar phase I study demonstrated low toxicity from everolimus, temozolomide and radiation in newly diagnosed glioblastoma therapy, [86] and as such a randomized phase II trial is ongoing (ClinicalTrials.gov NCT01062399). In both newly diagnosed and recurrent glioblastoma, a phase I study of temozolomide and everolimus showed low toxicity, with the caveat that enzyme-inducing antiseizure medications should be stopped with this drug due to increased clearance [87]. In a phase II study in newly diagnosed glioblastoma patients, concurrent radiation, temozolomide and bevacizumab were followed by adjuvant bevacizumab and everolimus [88]. The study was not powered to detect everolimus effect alone, but rather focused on PFS improvement with this combination in comparison with standard radiation and temozolomide, which was positive [88].

Temsirolimus, a third mTOR inhibitor, has been also studied in both newly diagnosed and recurrent glioblastoma. A phase II study of temsirolimus monotherapy showed modest radiographic improvement in about one-third of recurrent glioblastoma patients, with significantly longer time to progression compared to the two-thirds of patients who did not respond [89]. Also noted here was a correlation between responders and pretreatment levels of p70s6 tumor levels, suggesting a potential biomarker for treatment-specific response [89]. A second phase II study of temsirolimus monotherapy for recurrent glioblastoma showed early disease stability in about half of patients, but no durable response [90]. Further, in a phase II combination study with bevacizumab, no additional clinical efficacy was seen from temsirolimus above bevacizumab therapy alone [17]. A phase I/II trial combining temsirolimus with sorafenib for recurrent glioblastoma was not well tolerated and showed minimal antitumor activity [31]. In a study of temsirolimus with temozolomide and radiation in newly diagnosed glioblastoma, significant toxicity was seen with multiple grade 4 infections and immunosuppression, and minimal information was ascertained in regard to the antitumor effect of the combination [91].

Ridaforolimus, another mTOR inhibitor, showed evidence of crossing the BBB into tumor tissue, as well as decreasing mTOR activity as reflected by indirect measurement of decreased phospho-S6 levels. Unfortunately, these pharmacodynamic changes were not associated with any therapeutic benefit [92].

Although there has been significant interest in inhibiting the mTOR pathway, it is clear that inhibition of mTORC1 alone is insufficient, in part due to loss of the feedback inhibition on AKT [84]. Agents that target both mTORC1 and mTORC2 may have greater therapeutic potential and studies with agents such as INK128 (also known as MLN0128), CC115, CC223 are in progress (ClinicalTrials.gov NCT02133183, NCT01353625, NCT01177397).

9 RAS/RAF/MEK/ERK

Signaling through the RAS pathway, most commonly activated by EGFR cell-surface ligand or by inactivation of the *NF1* gene, activates downstream kinases RAF, then Mitogen-activated Erk Kinase (MEK), and finally Extracellular Signal-Regulated Kinase (ERK), an activator of transcription factors and protein translation, and represents a potential target in glioblastoma treatment.

Tipifarnib, a farnesyltransferase inhibitor shown to reduce signaling through this pathway, has been evaluated in several glioblastoma trials. The drug was well tolerated in phase I studies of newly diagnosed glioblastoma patients [93, 94]. However, a phase II study in newly diagnosed glioblastoma patients did not show significant benefit when given after resection and before radiation (in an era before concurrent chemotherapy with temozolomide) [95]. In recurrent high-grade glioma, tipifarnib showed minimal activity with an average 6-month PFS of 12 %, but the investigators noted significantly better outcomes among patients not receiving enzyme-inducing seizure medications [96]. Studies with sorafenib, a weak RAF inhibitor, have been uniformly disappointing.

There are now numerous RAF, MEK, and even ERK inhibitors in clinical trials. To date very few have been evaluated in glioblastoma patients because of poor penetration across the BBB. One ongoing trial evaluates the combination of the RAF inhibitor, dabrafenib, with the MEK inhibitor, trametanib, in recurrent gliomas with BRAFv600E mutations (ClincalTrials.gov ID NCT02034110).

10 Promyelocytic Leukemia (PML)

Resistance pathways for mTOR blockade are an ongoing source of research. The promyelocytic leukemia (PML) gene is a pleiotropic tumor suppressor gene that produces a nuclear protein complex by the same name, promoting cancer senescence and homeostasis [97]. Initially found in leukemia, this protein complex interacts with the PI3K pathway at many levels, including opposition to AKT signaling and decreasing mTOR activity through parallel signaling pathways [98, 99]. Arsenic trioxide has been shown to induce degradation of PML, and concurrent treatment with this compound and mTOR inhibitors has shown positive effects in vitro [100] and clinical trials with this combination in patients with recurrent glioblastomas are planned. To date, the only reported clinical trial of arsenic trioxide in high-grade gliomas was a phase I study, combined with temozolomide and radiation, demonstrating acceptable toxicity and a radiographic response in 35 % of patients and a promising 37-month overall survival [101]. As such, a phase II study of this combination is also under way (ClinicalTrials.gov NCT00275067).

11 Isocitrate Dehydrogenase-1 and 2 (IDH-1 and 2)

The Warburg effect, studied since in the 1920s, describes the use of anaerobic glycolysis by tumors even in the presence of adequate oxygenation, resulting in generation of fewer ATP molecules, but increased production of other molecules required for tumor growth [102]. Many oncogenes both promote tumor growth and also profoundly affect metabolic activity [103]. Two broad categories of oncogene-associated metabolic effects include pathway-associated enhanced glycolysis, as in the case of PI3K/AKT/mTOR, and direct oncogenic mutations in metabolic enzymes [103]. This second category is best exemplified by isocitrate dehydrogenase-1 (IDH-1). In recent tumor sequencing studies, IDH-1 mutations have been commonly identified in gliomas which are mostly low grade and have a relatively good prognosis [104, 105]. The most common mutation in IDH-1 is arginine to histidine at position 132 (R132H) [105]. This leads to a gain of function mutation in IDH-1, promoting an aberrant metabolic byproduct of 2-hydroxyglutarate (2HG) [106]. Mutation in IDH-1 has been identified commonly in approximately 60–70 % of grade II and III gliomas, as well as most secondary glioblastomas, and is highly correlated with good prognosis [107–109].

Data regarding IDH-1 mutation is still fairly new, so there is limited targeted therapy research to date. One compound, AGI-5198, was identified to selectively inhibit IDH-1 R132H and thereby deplete 2HG production, and has been shown to slow tumor growth in vitro [110]. Further, genes associated with gliogenic differentiation showed less expression after treatment with AGI-5198 [110]. A similar compound, AG120, is currently in phase I study of IDH1-mutated solid tumors, including gliomas (ClinicalTrials.gov NCT02073994).

12 Histone Deacetylase (HDAC)

Histone acetylation is an important mechanism of control over DNA coiling and uncoiling, and thereby gene expression [111]. By inhibiting histone deacetylase (HDAC), gene transcription is disrupted which slows cell division and possibly leads to apoptosis. Vorinostat (SAHA), a second-generation HDAC inhibitor, has been studied in recurrent glioblastoma in a phase II monotherapy trial [112]. The trial showed only very modest single-agent activity with a median overall survival of 5.7 months but confirmed that vorinostat was able to effectively cross the BBB and increase acetylation of histones H2B, H3, and H4. Notably, thrombocytopenia was present in a fifth of patients. Later, a phase I study of vorinostat with temozolomide in recurrent glioblastoma was tolerated well overall, though thrombocytopenia and one related grade 5 hemorrhage were dose-limiting toxicities that defined the MTD in this study [113]. The ALLIANCE cooperative group and the Adult Brain Tumor Consortium recently completed a phase I/II trial of vorinostat in combination with radiotherapy and temozolomide in newly diagnosed glioblastoma patients, demonstrating acceptable tolerability, though the phase II efficacy information has not yet been published (ClinicalTrials.gov NCT00731731) [114]. Another phase I study in glioblastoma combined vorinostat with bevacizumab and irinotecan [115]. This study found the same MTD for vorinostat, though with less thrombocytopenia, and secondarily showed an improved progression-free survival and overall survival compared with vorinostat alone [115]. Phase II studies evaluating the combinations of bevacizumab and vorinostat or bevacizumab and panobinostat, another HDAC inhibitor, are ongoing (ClinicalTrials.gov NCT01266031, NCT00859222).

13 Proteasome

The proteasome is responsible for programmed breakdown of intracellular proteins. When inhibited, cell-cycle proteins become dysregulated and apoptosis ensues. One proteasome inhibitor, bortezomib, has been evaluated in high-grade gliomas. A phase I clinical trial of bortezomib monotherapy for recurrent high-grade gliomas showed partial responses in only two of 66 patients [116]. In combination with temozolomide and radiation therapy, another phase I study showed bortezomib was a safe addition to this regimen and lead to a 15-month overall survival for high-grade glioma patients [117]. A phase II combination study of vorinostat and bortezomib was closed early when no patients had a 6-month progression-free survival [118]. The limited penetration of bortezomib across the BBB likely reduces potential antitumor activity.

14 Microtubule

Microtubules, found in the cytoplasm, are a key component of the cytoskeleton and provide an infrastructure for cellular functions such as mitosis and movement of secretory vesicles and organelles. Microtubule-stabilizing drugs, therefore, prevent the normal breakdown of cytoskeletal components during mitosis, and thereby halt cell division. Paclitaxel, a well-established microtubule-stabilizing chemotherapy, has been evaluated in high-grade gliomas with limited success. In one dose-escalation study for recurrent high-grade gliomas, 35 % of patients had stable or improved disease with paclitaxel monotherapy, though toxicity was quite high [119]. Another study in recurrent high-grade gliomas modified paclitaxel doses based on concurrent enzyme-inducing AEDs, but no objective responses were seen [120].

Conjugated paclitaxel and L-glutamic acid has improved water solubility, and has also been evaluated in a phase I study combined with temozolomide and radiation for newly diagnosed glioblastoma. Here, hematologic toxicity was profound and prolonged, making the combination unsafe overall [99]. To further improve tumor delivery of paclitaxel, and thereby reduce the overall dose necessary, ANG1005 (previously GRN1005) was developed. This is a conjugate of paclitaxel and Angiopep-2, which is a proprietary peptide sequence that crosses the BBB through targeting the LDL receptor-related protein 1. A phase I study of this drug showed good drug delivery to the tumor with a similar toxicity profile to paclitaxel [121], and a phase II study was recommended at the determined MTD, which is ongoing (ClinicalTrials.gov NCT01967810).

15 Summary

Preclinical advances in the molecular biology of gliomas have led to the development of many targeted chemotherapeutic approaches for the treatment of glioblastoma. Despite this progress, several challenges remain steadfastly ahead of broadly applicable patient benefit. First, poor CNS penetration of chemotherapeutics remains at the forefront of translational difficulties. Many trials are now including a surgical component to evaluate for drug tumor penetration, as well as on-target molecular efficacy of new agents. Second, the redundancy of signaling pathways, as well as coactivation of multiple RTK pathways in glioblastoma, is prohibitive for single-agent chemotherapy success. Focusing on multiple pathway blockade, or final common pathways, may be a useful consideration to overcome this challenge. Finally, the genetic heterogeneity among glioblastomas, a continually evolving landscape, underscores the importance of prospective tumor genotyping prior to trial enrollment, in order to best understand potential successes.

Although glioblastoma remains an incurable disease, with unacceptably poor prognosis, the advances in targeted therapies reviewed here provide a framework for future success. Combined treatment strategies and individualized regimens may well hold the key to increasing PFS and OS.

References

1. Wen PY, Kesari S (2008) Malignant gliomas in adults. N Engl J Med 359(5):492–507
2. Stupp R, Mason WP, van den Bent MJ et al (2005) Radiotherapy plus concomitant and adjuvant temozolomide for glioblastoma. N Engl J Med 352(10):987–996
3. Vredenburgh JJ, Desjardins A, Herndon JE 2nd et al (2007) Phase II trial of bevacizumab and irinotecan in recurrent malignant glioma. Clin Cancer Res Off J Am Assoc Cancer Res 13(4):1253–1259
4. Vredenburgh JJ, Desjardins A, Herndon JE 2nd et al (2007) Bevacizumab plus irinotecan in recurrent glioblastoma multiforme. J Clin Oncol Off J Am Soc Clin Oncol 25(30):4722–4729
5. Friedman HS, Prados MD, Wen PY et al (2009) Bevacizumab alone and in combination with irinotecan in recurrent glioblastoma. J Clin Oncol Off J Am Soc Clin Oncol 27 (28):4733–4740
6. Kreisl TN, Kim L, Moore K et al (2009) Phase II trial of single-agent bevacizumab followed by bevacizumab plus irinotecan at tumor progression in recurrent glioblastoma. J Clin Oncol Off J Am Soc Clin Oncol 27(5):740–745
7. Cohen MH, Shen YL, Keegan P, Pazdur R (2009) FDA drug approval summary: bevacizumab (Avastin) as treatment of recurrent glioblastoma multiforme. Oncologist 14 (11):1131–1138
8. Chinot OL, Wick W, Mason W et al (2014) Bevacizumab plus radiotherapy-temozolomide for newly diagnosed glioblastoma. N Engl J Med 370(8):709–722
9. Gilbert MR, Dignam JJ, Armstrong TS et al (2014) A randomized trial of bevacizumab for newly diagnosed glioblastoma. N Engl J Med 370(8):699–708
10. Arrillaga-Romany I, Reardon DA, Wen PY (2014) Current status of antiangiogenic therapies for glioblastomas. Expert Opin Investig Drugs 23(2):199–210
11. Moller S, Grunnet K, Hansen S et al (2012) A phase II trial with bevacizumab and irinotecan for patients with primary brain tumors and progression after standard therapy. Acta Oncol 51 (6):797–804
12. Hasselbalch B, Lassen U, Hansen S et al (2010) Cetuximab, bevacizumab, and irinotecan for patients with primary glioblastoma and progression after radiation therapy and temozolomide: a phase II trial. Neuro-oncology 12(5):508–516
13. Reardon DA, Desjardins A, Peters KB et al (2012) Phase II study of carboplatin, irinotecan, and bevacizumab for bevacizumab naive, recurrent glioblastoma. J Neurooncol 107(1):155–164
14. Galanis E, Anderson SK, Lafky JM et al (2013) Phase II study of bevacizumab in combination with sorafenib in recurrent glioblastoma (N0776): a north central cancer treatment group trial. Clin Cancer Res Off J Am Assoc Cancer Res 19(17):4816–4823
15. Desjardins A, Reardon DA, Coan A et al (2012) Bevacizumab and daily temozolomide for recurrent glioblastoma. Cancer 118(5):1302–1312
16. Sathornsumetee S, Desjardins A, Vredenburgh JJ et al (2010) Phase II trial of bevacizumab and erlotinib in patients with recurrent malignant glioma. Neuro-oncology 12(12):1300–1310
17. Lassen U, Sorensen M, Gaziel TB, Hasselbalch B, Poulsen HS (2013) Phase II study of bevacizumab and temsirolimus combination therapy for recurrent glioblastoma multiforme. Anticancer Res 33(4):1657–1660
18. Reardon DA, Desjardins A, Vredenburgh JJ et al (2009) Metronomic chemotherapy with daily, oral etoposide plus bevacizumab for recurrent malignant glioma: a phase II study. Br J Cancer 101(12):1986–1994
19. Soffietti R, Trevisan E, Bertero L et al (2014) Bevacizumab and fotemustine for recurrent glioblastoma: a phase II study of AINO (Italian Association of Neuro-Oncology). J Neurooncol 116(3):533–541
20. Reardon DA, Turner S, Peters KB et al (2011) A review of VEGF/VEGFR-targeted therapeutics for recurrent glioblastoma. J Natl Compr Cancer Netw JNCCN 9(4):414–427

21. de Groot JF, Lamborn KR, Chang SM et al (2011) Phase II study of aflibercept in recurrent malignant glioma: a North American brain tumor consortium study. J Clin Oncol 29 (19):2689–2695
22. Eliceiri BP, Cheresh DA (2000) Role of alpha v integrins during angiogenesis. Cancer J 6 (Suppl 3):S245–S249
23. Desgrosellier JS, Cheresh DA (2010) Integrins in cancer: biological implications and therapeutic opportunities. Nat Rev Cancer 10(1):9–22
24. Nabors LB, Mikkelsen T, Rosenfeld SS et al (2007) Phase I and correlative biology study of cilengitide in patients with recurrent malignant glioma. J Clin Oncol Off J Am Soc Clin Oncol 25(13):1651–1657
25. Reardon DA, Fink KL, Mikkelsen T et al (2008) Randomized phase II study of cilengitide, an integrin-targeting arginine-glycine-aspartic acid peptide, in recurrent glioblastoma multiforme. J Clin Oncol Off J Am Soc Clin Oncol 26(34):5610–5617
26. Gilbert MR, Kuhn J, Lamborn KR et al (2012) Cilengitide in patients with recurrent glioblastoma: the results of NABTC 03-02, a phase II trial with measures of treatment delivery. J Neurooncol 106(1):147–153
27. Nabors LB, Mikkelsen T, Hegi ME et al (2012) A safety run-in and randomized phase 2 study of cilengitide combined with chemoradiation for newly diagnosed glioblastoma (NABTT 0306). Cancer 118(22):5601–5607
28. Stupp R, Hegi ME, Neyns B et al (2010) Phase I/IIa study of cilengitide and temozolomide with concomitant radiotherapy followed by cilengitide and temozolomide maintenance therapy in patients with newly diagnosed glioblastoma. J Clin Oncol Off J Am Soc Clin Oncol 28(16):2712–2718
29. Stupp R, Hegi M, Gorlia T, Erridge S, Grujicic D et al (2013) Cilengitide combined with standard treatment for patients with newly diagnosed glioblastoma and methylated O6-methylguanine-DNA methyltransferase (MGMT) gene promoter: Key results of the multicenter, randomized, open-label, controlled, phase III CENTRIC study. J Clin Oncol Off J Am Soc Clin Oncol 31(18 Suppl), Abstract number LBA2009
30. Nabors L, Fink K, Mikkelsen T, Grujicic D, Tarnawski R et al. (2013) Cilengitide in combination with standard treatment for patients with newly diagnosed glioblastoma with unmethylated O6-methylguanine-DNA methyltransferase (MGMT) gene promoter: key results of the open-label, controlled, randomized phase II CORE study. Neuro-oncology 15 (Suppl 3):iii75–iii84
31. Cancer Genome Atlas Research N. (2008) Comprehensive genomic characterization defines human glioblastoma genes and core pathways. Nature 455(7216):1061–1068
32. Batchelor TT, Duda DG, di Tomaso E et al (2010) Phase II study of cediranib, an oral pan-vascular endothelial growth factor receptor tyrosine kinase inhibitor, in patients with recurrent glioblastoma. J Clin Oncol Off J Am Soc Clin Oncol 28(17):2817–2823
33. Batchelor TT, Mulholland P, Neyns B et al (2013) Phase III randomized trial comparing the efficacy of cediranib as monotherapy, and in combination with lomustine, versus lomustine alone in patients with recurrent glioblastoma. J Clin Oncol Off J Am Soc Clin Oncol 31 (26):3212–3218
34. Batchelor TT, Gerstner ER, Emblem KE et al (2013) Improved tumor oxygenation and survival in glioblastoma patients who show increased blood perfusion after cediranib and chemoradiation. Proc Natl Acad Sci USA 110(47):19059–19064
35. Kreisl TN, McNeill KA, Sul J, Iwamoto FM, Shih J, Fine HA (2012) A phase I/II trial of vandetanib for patients with recurrent malignant glioma. Neuro-oncology 14(12):1519–1526
36. Reardon DA, Vredenburgh JJ, Desjardins A et al (2011) Effect of CYP3A-inducing anti-epileptics on sorafenib exposure: results of a phase II study of sorafenib plus daily temozolomide in adults with recurrent glioblastoma. J Neurooncol 101(1):57–66
37. Zustovich F, Landi L, Lombardi G et al (2013) Sorafenib plus daily low-dose temozolomide for relapsed glioblastoma: a phase II study. Anticancer Res 33(8):3487–3494

38. Peereboom DM, Ahluwalia MS, Ye X et al (2013) NABTT 0502: a phase II and pharmacokinetic study of erlotinib and sorafenib for patients with progressive or recurrent glioblastoma multiforme. Neuro-oncology 15(4):490–496
39. Hainsworth JD, Ervin T, Friedman E et al (2010) Concurrent radiotherapy and temozolomide followed by temozolomide and sorafenib in the first-line treatment of patients with glioblastoma multiforme. Cancer 116(15):3663–3669
40. Lee EQ, Kuhn J, Lamborn KR et al (2012) Phase I/II study of sorafenib in combination with temsirolimus for recurrent glioblastoma or gliosarcoma: North American Brain Tumor Consortium study 05-02. Neuro-oncology 14(12):1511–1518
41. Iwamoto FM, Lamborn KR, Robins HI et al (2010) Phase II trial of pazopanib (GW786034), an oral multi-targeted angiogenesis inhibitor, for adults with recurrent glioblastoma (North American Brain Tumor Consortium Study 06-02). Neuro-oncology 12(8):855–861
42. Reardon DA, Groves MD, Wen PY et al (2013) A phase I/II trial of pazopanib in combination with lapatinib in adult patients with relapsed malignant glioma. Clin Cancer Res 19(4):900–908
43. Rampling R, Sanson M, Gorlia T et al (2012) A phase I study of LY317615 (enzastaurin) and temozolomide in patients with gliomas (EORTC trial 26054). Neuro-oncology 14 (3):344–350
44. Wick W, Puduvalli VK, Chamberlain MC et al (2010) Phase III study of enzastaurin compared with lomustine in the treatment of recurrent intracranial glioblastoma. J Clin Oncol Off J Am Soc Clin Oncol 28(7):1168–1174
45. Goldlust SA, Cavaliere R, Newton HB et al (2012) Bevacizumab for glioblastoma refractory to vascular endothelial growth factor receptor inhibitors. J Neurooncol 107(2):407–411
46. Scott BJ, Quant EC, McNamara MB, Ryg PA, Batchelor TT, Wen PY (2010) Bevacizumab salvage therapy following progression in high-grade glioma patients treated with VEGF receptor tyrosine kinase inhibitors. Neuro-oncology 12(6):603–607
47. Ohgaki H, Dessen P, Jourde B et al (2004) Genetic pathways to glioblastoma: a population-based study. Cancer Res 64(19):6892–6899
48. Shinojima N, Tada K, Shiraishi S et al (2003) Prognostic value of epidermal growth factor receptor in patients with glioblastoma multiforme. Cancer Res 63(20):6962–6970
49. Wong AJ, Bigner SH, Bigner DD, Kinzler KW, Hamilton SR, Vogelstein B (1987) Increased expression of the epidermal growth factor receptor gene in malignant gliomas is invariably associated with gene amplification. Proc Natl Acad Sci USA 84(19):6899–6903
50. van den Bent MJ, Brandes AA, Rampling R et al (2009) Randomized phase II trial of erlotinib versus temozolomide or carmustine in recurrent glioblastoma: EORTC brain tumor group study 26034. J Clin Oncol Off J Am Soc Clin Oncol 27(8):1268–1274
51. D'Alessandris QG, Montano N, Cenci T et al (2013) Targeted therapy with bevacizumab and erlotinib tailored to the molecular profile of patients with recurrent glioblastoma. Preliminary experience. Acta Neurochi 155(1):33–40
52. Wen PY, Chang SM, Lamborn KR et al (2014) Phase I/II study of erlotinib and temsirolimus for patients with recurrent malignant gliomas: North American Brain Tumor Consortium trial 04-02. Neuro-oncology
53. Nghiemphu PL, Lai A, Green RM, Reardon DA, Cloughesy T (2012) A dose escalation trial for the combination of erlotinib and sirolimus for recurrent malignant gliomas. J Neurooncol 110(2):245–250
54. Reardon DA, Vredenburgh JJ, Desjardins A et al (2012) Phase 1 trial of dasatinib plus erlotinib in adults with recurrent malignant glioma. J Neurooncol 108(3):499–506
55. Prados MD, Chang SM, Butowski N et al (2009) Phase II study of erlotinib plus temozolomide during and after radiation therapy in patients with newly diagnosed glioblastoma multiforme or gliosarcoma. J Clin Oncol Off J Am Soc Clin Oncol 27 (4):579–584
56. Brown PD, Krishnan S, Sarkaria JN et al (2008) Phase I/II trial of erlotinib and temozolomide with radiation therapy in the treatment of newly diagnosed glioblastoma

multiforme: North Central Cancer Treatment Group Study N0177. J Clin Oncol Off J Am Soc Clin Oncol 26(34):5603–5609

57. Haas-Kogan DA, Prados MD, Tihan T et al (2005) Epidermal growth factor receptor, protein kinase B/Akt, and glioma response to erlotinib. J Natl Cancer Inst 97(12):880–887
58. Yung WK, Vredenburgh JJ, Cloughesy TF et al (2010) Safety and efficacy of erlotinib in first-relapse glioblastoma: a phase II open-label study. Neuro-oncology 12(10):1061–1070
59. Mellinghoff IK, Wang MY, Vivanco I et al (2005) Molecular determinants of the response of glioblastomas to EGFR kinase inhibitors. N Engl J Med 353(19):2012–2024
60. Gallego O, Cuatrecasas M, Benavides M et al (2014) Efficacy of erlotinib in patients with relapsed gliobastoma multiforme who expressed EGFRVIII and PTEN determined by immunohistochemistry. J Neurooncology 116(2):413–419
61. Rich JN, Reardon DA, Peery T et al (2004) Phase II trial of gefitinib in recurrent glioblastoma. J Clin Oncol 22(1):133–142
62. Kreisl TN, Lassman AB, Mischel PS et al (2009) A pilot study of everolimus and gefitinib in the treatment of recurrent glioblastoma (GBM). J Neurooncol 92(1):99–105
63. Rich JN, Rasheed BK, Yan H. (2004) EGFR mutations and sensitivity to gefitinib. N Engl J Med 351(12):1260–1261 (author reply 1260–1261)
64. Thiessen B, Stewart C, Tsao M et al (2010) A phase I/II trial of GW572016 (lapatinib) in recurrent glioblastoma multiforme: clinical outcomes, pharmacokinetics and molecular correlation. Cancer Chemother Pharmacol 65(2):353–361
65. Karavasilis V, Kotoula V, Pentheroudakis G et al (2013) A phase I study of temozolomide and lapatinib combination in patients with recurrent high-grade gliomas. J Neurol 260 (6):1469–1480
66. Vivanco I, Robins HI, Rohle D et al (2012) Differential sensitivity of glioma-versus lung cancer-specific EGFR mutations to EGFR kinase inhibitors. Cancer Discovery 2(5):458–471
67. Brennan CW, Verhaak RG, McKenna A et al (2013) The somatic genomic landscape of glioblastoma. Cell 155(2):462–477
68. Demetri GD, von Mehren M, Blanke CD et al (2002) Efficacy and safety of imatinib mesylate in advanced gastrointestinal stromal tumors. N Engl J Med 347(7):472–480
69. O'Brien SG, Guilhot F, Larson RA et al (2003) Imatinib compared with interferon and low-dose cytarabine for newly diagnosed chronic-phase chronic myeloid leukemia. N Engl J Med 348(11):994–1004
70. Razis E, Selviaridis P, Labropoulos S et al (2009) Phase II study of neoadjuvant imatinib in glioblastoma: evaluation of clinical and molecular effects of the treatment. Clin Cancer Res Off J Am Assoc Cancer Res 15(19):6258–6266
71. Raymond E, Brandes AA, Dittrich C et al (2008) Phase II study of imatinib in patients with recurrent gliomas of various histologies: a European Organisation for Research and Treatment of Cancer Brain Tumor Group Study. J Clin Oncol Off J Am Soc Clin Oncol 26 (28):4659–4665
72. Reardon DA, Dresemann G, Taillibert S et al (2009) Multicentre phase II studies evaluating imatinib plus hydroxyurea in patients with progressive glioblastoma. Br J Cancer 101 (12):1995–2004
73. Wen PY, Yung WK, Lamborn KR et al (2006) Phase I/II study of imatinib mesylate for recurrent malignant gliomas: North American Brain Tumor Consortium Study 99-08. Clin Cancer Res 12(16):4899–4907
74. Desjardins A, Quinn JA, Vredenburgh JJ et al (2007) Phase II study of imatinib mesylate and hydroxyurea for recurrent grade III malignant gliomas. J Neurooncol 83(1):53–60
75. Reardon DA, Egorin MJ, Quinn JA et al (2005) Phase II study of imatinib mesylate plus hydroxyurea in adults with recurrent glioblastoma multiforme. J Clin Oncol Off J Am Soc Clin Oncol 23(36):9359–9368
76. Franceschi E, Stupp R, van den Bent MJ et al (2012) EORTC 26083 phase I/II trial of dasatinib in combination with CCNU in patients with recurrent glioblastoma. Neuro-oncology 14(12):1503–1510

77. Lassman AB, Wang M, Gilbert M, Aldape K, Beumer JH, et al. (2011) Phase II trial of dasatinib in target selected patients with recurrent glioblastoma (RTOG 0627). Neuro-oncology 13(Supple 3), Abstract number 102
78. Lu-Emerson C, Norden AD, Drappatz J et al (2011) Retrospective study of dasatinib for recurrent glioblastoma after bevacizumab failure. J Neurooncol 104(1):287–291
79. Wen PY, Lee EQ, Reardon DA, Ligon KL (2012) Alfred Yung WK. Current clinical development of PI3K pathway inhibitors in glioblastoma. Neuro-oncology 14(7):819–829
80. Chakravarti A, Zhai G, Suzuki Y et al (2004) The prognostic significance of phosphatidylinositol 3-kinase pathway activation in human gliomas. J Clin Oncol Off J Am Soc Clin Oncol 22(10):1926–1933
81. Bendell JC, Rodon J, Burris HA et al (2012) Phase I, dose-escalation study of BKM120, an oral pan-Class I PI3K inhibitor, in patients with advanced solid tumors. J Clin Oncol Off J Am Soc Clin Oncol 30(3):282–290
82. Wen P, Yung A, Mellinghoff IK et al. (2014) Phase II trial of phosphatidylinositol-3 kinase (PI3K) inhibitor buparlisib (BKM120) in recurrent glioblastoma. J Clin Oncol Off J Am Soc Clin Oncol 32(5 s), Abstract number 2019
83. Hong DS, Bowles DW, Falchook GS et al (2012) A multicenter phase I trial of PX-866, an oral irreversible phosphatidylinositol 3-kinase inhibitor, in patients with advanced solid tumors. Clin Cancer Res Off J Am Assoc Cancer Res 18(15):4173–4182
84. Cloughesy TF, Yoshimoto K, Nghiemphu P et al. (2008) Antitumor activity of rapamycin in a phase I trial for patients with recurrent PTEN-deficient glioblastoma. PLoS Med 5(1):e8
85. Sarkaria JN, Galanis E, Wu W et al (2011) North Central cancer treatment group phase I trial N057 K of everolimus (RAD001) and temozolomide in combination with radiation therapy in patients with newly diagnosed glioblastoma multiforme. Int J Radiat Oncol Biol Phys 81 (2):468–475
86. Chinnaiyan P, Won M, Wen PY et al (2013) RTOG 0913: a phase 1 study of daily everolimus (RAD001) in combination with radiation therapy and temozolomide in patients with newly diagnosed glioblastoma. Int J Radiat Oncol Biol Phys 86(5):880–884
87. Mason WP, Macneil M, Kavan P et al (2012) A phase I study of temozolomide and everolimus (RAD001) in patients with newly diagnosed and progressive glioblastoma either receiving or not receiving enzyme-inducing anticonvulsants: an NCIC CTG study. Invest New Drugs 30(6):2344–2351
88. Hainsworth JD, Shih KC, Shepard GC, Tillinghast GW, Brinker BT, Spigel DR (2012) Phase II study of concurrent radiation therapy, temozolomide, and bevacizumab followed by bevacizumab/everolimus as first-line treatment for patients with glioblastoma. Clin Adv Hematol Oncol H&O 10(4):240–246
89. Galanis E, Buckner JC, Maurer MJ et al (2005) Phase II trial of temsirolimus (CCI-779) in recurrent glioblastoma multiforme: a North Central Cancer Treatment Group Study. J Clin Oncol Off J Am S Clin Oncol 23(23):5294–5304
90. Chang SM, Wen P, Cloughesy T et al (2005) Phase II study of CCI-779 in patients with recurrent glioblastoma multiforme. Invest New Drugs 23(4):357–361
91. Sarkaria JN, Galanis E, Wu W et al (2010) Combination of temsirolimus (CCI-779) with chemoradiation in newly diagnosed glioblastoma multiforme (GBM) (NCCTG trial N027D) is associated with increased infectious risks. Clin Cancer Res Off J Am Assoc Cancer Res 16 (22):5573–5580
92. Reardon DA, Wen PY, Alfred Yung WK et al (2012) Ridaforolimus for patients with progressive or recurrent malignant glioma: a perisurgical, sequential, ascending-dose trial. Cancer Chemother Pharmacol 69(4):849–860
93. Nghiemphu PL, Wen PY, Lamborn KR et al (2011) A phase I trial of tipifarnib with radiation therapy, with and without temozolomide, for patients with newly diagnosed glioblastoma. Int J Radiat Oncol Biol Phys 81(5):1422–1427

94. Moyal EC, Laprie A, Delannes M et al (2007) Phase I trial of tipifarnib (R115777) concurrent with radiotherapy in patients with glioblastoma multiforme. Int J Radiat Oncol Biol Phys 68(5):1396–1401
95. Lustig R, Mikkelsen T, Lesser G et al (2008) Phase II preradiation R115777 (tipifarnib) in newly diagnosed GBM with residual enhancing disease. Neuro-oncology. 10(6):1004–1009
96. Cloughesy TF, Wen PY, Robins HI et al (2006) Phase II trial of tipifarnib in patients with recurrent malignant glioma either receiving or not receiving enzyme-inducing antiepileptic drugs: a North American Brain Tumor Consortium Study. J Clin Oncol Off J Am Soc Clin Oncol 24(22):3651–3656
97. Bernardi R, Pandolfi PP (2003) Role of PML and the PML-nuclear body in the control of programmed cell death. Oncogene 22(56):9048–9057
98. Trotman LC, Alimonti A, Scaglioni PP, Koutcher JA, Cordon-Cardo C (2006) Pandolfi PP. Identification of a tumour suppressor network opposing nuclear Akt function. Nature 441 (7092):523–527
99. Bernardi R, Scaglioni PP, Bergmann S, Horn HF, Vousden KH, Pandolfi PP (2004) PML regulates p53 stability by sequestering Mdm2 to the nucleolus. Nat Cell Biol 6(7):665–672
100. Iwanami A, Gini B, Zanca C et al (2013) PML mediates glioblastoma resistance to mammalian target of rapamycin (mTOR)-targeted therapies. Proc Natl Acad Sci USA 110 (11):4339–4344
101. Grimm SA, Marymont M, Chandler JP et al (2012) Phase I study of arsenic trioxide and temozolomide in combination with radiation therapy in patients with malignant gliomas. J Neurooncol 110(2):237–243
102. Warburg O (1956) On the origin of cancer cells. Science 123(3191):309–314
103. DeBerardinis RJ, Thompson CB (2012) Cellular metabolism and disease: what do metabolic outliers teach us? Cell 148(6):1132–1144
104. Yan H, Parsons DW, Jin G et al (2009) IDH1 and IDH2 mutations in gliomas. N Engl J Med 360(8):765–773
105. Parsons DW, Jones S, Zhang X et al (2008) An integrated genomic analysis of human glioblastoma multiforme. Science 321(5897):1807–1812
106. Dang L, White DW, Gross S et al (2009) Cancer-associated IDH1 mutations produce 2-hydroxyglutarate. Nature 462(7274):739–744
107. van den Bent MJ, Dubbink HJ, Marie Y et al (2010) IDH1 and IDH2 mutations are prognostic but not predictive for outcome in anaplastic oligodendroglial tumors: a report of the European organization for research and treatment of cancer brain tumor group. Clin Cancer Res Off J Am Assoc Cancer Res 16(5):1597–1604
108. Cheng HB, Yue W, Xie C, Zhang RY, Hu SS, Wang Z (2013) IDH1 mutation is associated with improved overall survival in patients with glioblastoma: a meta-analysis. Tumour Biol J Int Soc Oncodevelopmental Biol Med 34(6):3555–3559
109. Dahlrot RH, Kristensen BW, Hjelmborg J, Herrstedt J, Hansen S (2013) A population-based study of low-grade gliomas and mutated isocitrate dehydrogenase 1 (IDH1). J Neurooncol 114(3):309–317
110. Rohle D, Popovici-Muller J, Palaskas N et al (2013) An inhibitor of mutant IDH1 delays growth and promotes differentiation of glioma cells. Science 340(6132):626–630
111. Portela A, Esteller M (2010) Epigenetic modifications and human disease. Nat Biotechnol 28 (10):1057–1068
112. Galanis E, Jaeckle KA, Maurer MJ et al (2009) Phase II trial of vorinostat in recurrent glioblastoma multiforme: a north central cancer treatment group study. J Clin Oncol Off J Am Soc Clin Oncol 27(12):2052–2058
113. Lee EQ, Puduvalli VK, Reid JM et al (2012) Phase I study of vorinostat in combination with temozolomide in patients with high-grade gliomas: North American Brain Tumor Consortium Study 04-03. Clin Cancer Res Off J Am Assoc Cancer Res 18(21):6032–6039
114. Galanis E, Sarkaria JN, Anderson SK et al (2013) Phase I/II trial of vorinostat combined with temozolomide (TMZ) and radiation therapy (RT) for newly diagnosed glioblastoma (GBM)

(N0874-ABTC0902, Alliance): final results of the phase I trial. J Clin Oncol Off J Am Soc Clin Oncol 31(Suppl):Abstr 2046
115. Chinnaiyan P, Chowdhary S, Potthast L et al (2012) Phase I trial of vorinostat combined with bevacizumab and CPT-11 in recurrent glioblastoma. Neuro-oncology 14(1):93–100
116. Phuphanich S, Supko JG, Carson KA et al (2010) Phase 1 clinical trial of bortezomib in adults with recurrent malignant glioma. J Neurooncol 100(1):95–103
117. Kubicek GJ, Werner-Wasik M, Machtay M et al (2009) Phase I trial using proteasome inhibitor bortezomib and concurrent temozolomide and radiotherapy for central nervous system malignancies. Int J Radiat Oncol Biol Phys 74(2):433–439
118. Friday BB, Anderson SK, Buckner J et al (2012) Phase II trial of vorinostat in combination with bortezomib in recurrent glioblastoma: a North Central Cancer Treatment Group Study. Neuro-oncology. 14(2):215–221
119. Prados MD, Schold SC, Spence AM et al (1996) Phase II study of paclitaxel in patients with recurrent malignant glioma. J Clin Oncol Off J Am Soc Clin Oncol 14(8):2316–2321
120. Chang SM, Kuhn JG, Robins HI et al (2001) A Phase II study of paclitaxel in patients with recurrent malignant glioma using different doses depending upon the concomitant use of anticonvulsants: a North American brain tumor consortium report. Cancer 91(2):417–422
121. Drappatz J, Brenner A, Wong ET et al (2013) Phase I study of GRN1005 in recurrent malignant glioma. Clin Can Res Off J Am Assoc Cancer Res 19(6):1567–1576

Immunotherapy for Malignant Gliomas

Orin Bloch

Abstract Cancer immunotherapy aims to harness the innate ability of the immune system to recognize and destroy malignant cells. Immunotherapy for malignant gliomas is an emerging field that promises the possibility of highly specific and less toxic treatment compared to conventional chemotherapy. In addition, immunotherapy has the added benefit of sustained efficacy once immunologic memory is induced. Although there are numerous therapeutic agents that boost general immune function and facilitate improved antitumor immunity, to date, immunotherapy for gliomas has focused primarily on active vaccination against tumor-specific antigens. The results of numerous early phase clinical trials demonstrate promising results for vaccine therapy, but no therapy has yet proven to improve survival in a randomized, controlled trial. The major barrier to immunotherapy in malignant gliomas is tumor-induced immunosuppression. The mechanisms of immunosuppression are only now being elucidated, but clearly involve a combination of factors including regulatory T cells, tumor-associated PD-L1 expression, and CTLA-4 signaling. Immunomodulatory agents have been developed to combat these immunosuppressive factors and have demonstrated efficacy in other cancers. The future of glioma immunotherapy likely lies in a combination of active vaccination and immune checkpoint inhibition.

Keywords Glioma · Glioblastoma · Immunotherapy · Vaccine · CTLA-4 · PD-L1 · PD-1

Contents

O. Bloch (✉)
Department of Neurological Surgery, Northwestern University, Feinberg School of Medicine, 676 N. St. Clair Street, Suite 2210, Chicago, IL 60611, USA
e-mail: orin.bloch@northwestern.edu

J. Raizer and A. Parsa (eds.), *Current Understanding and Treatment of Gliomas*, Cancer Treatment and Research 163, DOI 10.1007/978-3-319-12048-5_9

1 Cancer Immunotherapy

Under normal conditions, the immune system scavenges the body not only for infection, but also for mutations and malignant degeneration of its own cells. Immune surveillance and immunoediting keeps mutations in check, preventing true malignancy before it begins [1]. Most systemic cancers arise only when neoplastic cells escape immune control [2]. It is well recognized that patients with defects in normal immune function are prone to developing multiple malignancies [3].

Cancer immunotherapy is broadly defined as any therapy that utilizes the immune system to destroy malignant cells, thereby reestablishing immune control of tumor growth [4]. Immunotherapy can be passive or active. Passive immunotherapy employs administration of antibodies or activated immune cells that target a specific antigen expressed by the tumor. For example, monoclonal antibodies such as trastuzumab target the HER2/neu receptor in breast cancer leading to signaling blockade and arrest of tumor proliferation [5]. Adoptive transfer of modified chimeric antigen receptor (CAR) T cells utilizes immune cells that are generated and expanded ex vivo to attack and destroy malignancies [6]. These passive immunotherapy strategies rely on introduction of exogenous immune factors not replicated by the patient's own immune system. Their limitation, like any chemotherapeutic agent, is that efficacy only lasts as long as the agent is given. In addition, they target a single tumor marker, selecting for growth of tumor cells that do not express this marker. In contrast, active immunotherapy employs the immune system's innate response to the tumor. Active immunotherapy may consist of immunomodulatory agents that boost already established but insufficient immune responses, or may involve vaccination against tumor antigens to educate the immune system to recognize new tumor targets [7]. Active immunotherapy may have a single or multiple antigenic targets, and can have sustained efficacy long after the therapy is given.

The primary effector of the innate immune response to malignancy is the cytolytic $CD8^+$ T cell (CTL) [8]. Clonal populations of CTLs with T cell receptors that specifically recognize tumor antigens can bind to class I major histocompatibility complexes (MHC) expressing the antigen on the tumor surface. This results in tumor cell destruction through a variety of mechanisms [9]. Education of tumor-specific CTLs begins in the peripheral circulation, where antigen presenting cells

(APC) displaying tumor-specific peptides encounter naïve T cells. When this binding occurs in the presence of the appropriate costimulatory factors, clonal expansion and activation of tumor-specific T cells results.

Some immunomodulatory agents nonspecifically enhance the natural process of T cell education and activation/expansion to boost the innate immune response. Agents such as interleukin-2 (IL-2) facilitate clonal expansion of T cells once appropriate binding to the APC occurs [10]. IL-2 immunotherapy has shown significant promise for the treatment of renal cell carcinoma and melanoma [11, 12]. Other agents such as interferons and toll-like receptor (TLR) agonists, nonspecifically activate proinflammatory pathways in multiple immune cells, resulting in increased T cell activity [13]. The latest trend in immunotherapy has been modulation of immune checkpoints intended to prevent overactivation of the immune response and autoimmunity [14]. Agents such as ipilumumab that inhibit CTLA-4 signaling appear to boost T cell-mediated immunity and have shown significant responses in patients with melanoma [15]. An alternative approach to nonspecifically boosting immunity, is to direct an immune response against a specific tumor antigen by vaccination. The first cancer vaccine, which utilized dendritic cells (DCs) pulsed with antigenic peptides targeting prostate, was approved by the FDA in 2010 [16]. Tumor vaccines can be generated to target tumor-specific markers, and have the added benefit of generating immunologic memory for sustained efficacy even after the vaccination period is over.

1.1 Immunotherapy for Gliomas

Active immunotherapy relies on systemic exposure to tumor-specific antigens and sufficient costimulus for activation of CTLs. For most systemic cancers, recognition of tumor antigens occurs naturally as part of routine immunoediting [17]. In contrast, the brain is a relatively immune-privileged space, protected behind the blood—brain barrier (BBB). Rather than being scavenged by DCs, foreign antigen recognition in the brain is usually left up to resident microglia and astrocytes that express TLRs [18, 19]. Only once an inflammatory response is initiated and cytokines are produced by resident cells, does the BBB become permeable to peripheral immune cells [20]. High-grade gliomas, associated with significant necrosis and inflammation, are known to be infiltrated by peripheral immune effector cells [21]. The majority of immune cells in high-grade tumors are macrophages, with T cells representing only 5–10 % of infiltrating cells [22]. Therefore, unlike most systemic tumors that are recognized by the immune system prior to escaping immune surveillance, glial tumor antigens may not be recognized by the peripheral immune system until the tumors have substantially progressed and become highly inflammatory. Even once high-grade tumors are infiltrated by immune effectors, it is unclear how well tumor antigens are presented by APCs in circulation. Therefore, the primary modality of immunotherapy for gliomas to date has been active tumor vaccination rather than the use of immunomodulatory agents.

Vaccination ensures that the immune system is educated against tumor-specific peptides rather than nonspecifically activated.

2 Glioma Vaccines

Numerous vaccines targeting glioblastoma (GBM) have been tested in clinical trials (Table 1). The various vaccines differ in the antigenic peptides that they target and the method by which the antigen is delivered to the immune system. Ultimately, a successful vaccine must deliver a tumor-specific peptide(s) to the patient's APCs such that the peptide is displayed on class I MHC and presented to naïve T cells in circulation for education and clonal expansion. This can be accomplished by delivering tumor cell fragments or naked peptides systemically along with an immune adjuvant that stimulates uptake by circulating APCs and T cell proliferation. Alternatively, DCs can be extracted by plasmapheresis and pulsed with tumor antigens ex vivo. The antigen presenting DCs can then be reintroduced into circulation to activate T cells. Finally, antigens can be delivered to DCs in circulation using specialized antigen carriers such as heat shock proteins (HSP). Each of these approaches has been used as a vaccine modality for GBM in a clinical trial.

2.1 Peptide Vaccines

Systemic delivery of tumor-specific peptides or cell fragments can be used to educate and activate CTLs through uptake and presentation by dermal APCs. The process of uptake and expression of the antigenic peptides is enhanced by conjugating them to immune stimulants, such as keyhole limpet hemocyanin (KLH), and/or simultaneously administering leukocyte growth factors, such as GM-CSF or IL-2. The key to this approach is delivering peptides that are significantly expressed and highly specific for the tumor. Vaccines can be created by selecting antigenic target(s) and generating synthetic peptides, by extracting specific peptides from tumor lysates, or by nonspecifically delivering tumor cell lysates with a variety of antigenic peptides.

The most investigated target of a specific peptide vaccine in GBM is the tumor variant epidermal growth factor receptor (EGFRvIII). Amplification and overactivation of EGFR is a common mutation seen in GBM [23]. Approximately 30–40 % of GBM patients express an aberrant receptor, EGFRvIII, which remains constitutively active regardless of ligand binding, driving cell activity [24]. EGFRvIII is only expressed by GBM cells, making it an ideal target for vaccine therapy. A peptide vaccine containing a 14 amino acid antigenic sequence for EGFRvIII conjugated to KHL (rindopepimut) has been studied in phase II and III trials for newly diagnosed and recurrent GBM [25]. In the ACTIVATE trial, 18 patients received the vaccine and concurrent GM-CSF for newly diagnosed GBM following

Table 1 Vaccine clinical trials for glioblastoma

Trial	Vaccine	Type	Phase	Experimental design	N	PFS (mo)	OS (mo)
NCT00612001 [32]		DC	I	Autologous DC + selected glioma antigens	6	9.6	18.1
NCT00846456 [59]		DC	I/II	Autologous DC transfected with GSC mRNA for GBM	7	22.3	24.4
NCT00323115 [60]		DC	II	Autologous DC + tumor lysate for new GBM by intranodal injection	10	9.5	28
NCT00576641 [31]	ICT-107	DC	I	Autologous DC + GSC peptides for new GBM	17	16.9	38.4
NCT00068510 [33]	DCVax-L	DC	I	Autologous DC + tumor lysate for malignant glioma	28	18.1	34.4
NCT00576537 [34]		DC	II	Autologous DC + tumor lysate for malignant glioma	32	8	18
NCT01280552 [61]	ICT-107	DC	IIb	Randomized, placebo-controlled DC + selected peptides for new GBM	81	11.2	18.3
NCT02049489	ICT-121	DC	I	DC Vaccine against CD133 for recurrent GBM		Ongoing	
NCT02010606		DC	I	Autologous DC pulsed with allogenicglioma stem cell lysate for new and recurrent GBM		Ongoing	
NCT01957956		DC	I	Autologous DC + tumor lysate for new GBM		Ongoing	
NCT01808820		DC	I	Autologous DC + tumor lysate vaccine + imiquimod for HGG		Ongoing	
NCT00890032		DC	I	GSC mRNA loaded DC after surgery for recurrent GBM		Ongoing	
NCT00639639		DC	I	CMV pp65-LAMP mRNA loaded Dcfor new GBM		Ongoing	
NCT01204684		DC	II	Autologous DC + tumor lysate + Poly-ICLC for malignant glioma		Ongoing	
NCT00045968	DCVax-L	DC	III	Randomized, placebo-controlled DC + tumor lysate for new GBM		Ongoing	

(continued)

Table 1 (continued)

Trial	Vaccine	Type	Phase	Experimental design	N	PFS (mo)	OS (mo)
NCT00293423 [38]	HSPPC-96	HSP	II	Autologous HSP vaccine for recurrent GBM	41	5	10.5
NCT00905060 [39]	HSPPC-96	HSP	II	Autologous HSP vaccine for new GBM	46	16	23.3
NCT01814813	HSPPC-96	HSP	II	HSP vaccine + bev versus bev alone for recurrent GBM		Ongoing	
NCT00643097 [26]	PEP-3	Peptide	II	EGFRvIII vaccine + GM-CSF for new GBM - Part I (ACTIVATe)	18	12.3	20.4
NCT00643097 [26]	PEP-3	Peptide	II	EGFRvIII vaccine + GM-CSF for new GBM- Part 2 (ACT II)	22	15.3	20.5
NCT00458601 [62]	PEP-3	Peptide	II	EGFRvIII vaccine + GM-CSF for new GBM- Part 3 (ACT III)	65	12.3	21.8
NCT02149225	GAPVAC	Peptide	I	Personalized polypeptide vaccine + Poly-ICLC for new GBM		not open	
NCT01222221	IMA950	Peptide	I	Multivalent Peptide Vaccine + GM-CSF for new GBM		Ongoing	
NCT01250470	ISA-51	Peptide	I	Survivin peptide vaccine for malignant glioma		Ongoing	
NCT01854099	PEP-CMV	Peptide	I	CMV Antigen vaccine for new GBM		Withdrawn	
NCT01621542	WT2725	Peptide	I	WT peptide vaccine for advanced solid malignancies (including GBM)		Ongoing	
NCT01400672		Peptide	I	Allogenic BTIC cell line lysate + imiquimod for DIPG		Ongoing	
NCT00069940		Peptide	I	Telomerase peptide vaccine + GM-CSF for sarcomas or GBM		Ongoing	
NCT01920191	IMA950	Peptide	I/II	Multivalent peptide vaccine + Poly-ICLC + TMZ for new GBM		Ongoing	
NCT02078648	SL-701	Peptide	I/II	Multivalent peptide vaccine + imiquimod for recurrent GBM		Ongoing	
NCT01498328	PEP-3	Peptide	II	EGFRvIII vaccine + GM-CSF + BEV versus Placebo + BEV for recurrent GBM (ReACT)		Ongoing	
NCT01480479	PEP-3	Peptide	III	EGFRvIII vaccine + GM-CSF versus Placebo for new GBM- Part 3 (ACT IV)		Ongoing	

N number of patients, *PFS* progression-free survival (in months), *OS* overall survival (in months), *DC* dendritic cell, *HSP* heat shock protein, *GBM* glioblastoma, *GSC* glioma stem cell surgical resection and standard concurrent temozolomide chemotherapy and conformal radiotherapy (NCT00643097). The median progression-free survival (PFS) in the study was 12.3 months. In the ACT II trial, 22 patients received the vaccine after standard therapy and went on to adjuvant temozolomide therapy after progression (NCT00643097). Median PFS was 15.3 months and overall survival (OS) was 20.5 months [26]. The primary outcome measure in these trials was PFS, which faired favorably against historical control data from disease-matched patients with a median PFS of 6.4 months. These results led to the ACT III study, a phase II trial of the vaccine following surgery and chemoradiotherapy for newly diagnosed GBM, given concurrently with maintenance temozolomide (NCT00458601). The primary outcome for this trial was also PFS, with a median PFS of 12.3 months and a median OS of 21.8 months. A phase III trial of the EGFRvIII vaccine with adjuvant temozolomide versus placebo with temozolomide is currently ongoing (ACT IV; NCT01480479). Additionally, a phase II trial of the vaccine with bevacizumab versus bevacizumab alone for recurrent GBM in adults is ongoing (ReACT; NCT01498328).

In addition to EGFR, a number of other target proteins have been used to develop peptide vaccines for GBM. A Japanese phase II trial of a peptide vaccine targeting the Wilms Tumor (WT1) protein in recurrent gliomas demonstrated a median PFS of 5 months [27]. A phase I trial of a WT vaccine for advanced solid malignancies including GBM is now underway in the United States. Other phase I trials targeting a survivin peptide, CMV antigens, and telomerase are ongoing (see Table 1). The challenge for peptide vaccines with a single target is that their use is limited to patients who express the target. In the case of EGFRvIII, only 30–40 % of patients are eligible to receive the vaccine based on target protein expression. Furthermore, GBM is known to have significant heterogeneity in gene expression from cell to cell within the tumor [28]. Targeting a single protein may lead to eradication of all cells expressing that target, but other cells may survive, resulting in recurrence with selection for tumor that is not recognized by the immune response. This was demonstrated with the EGFRvIII peptide vaccine in the phase II trial [26]. All patients in the trial were histologically proven to have EGFRvIII expression at enrollment; however, of the 11 patients in the trial who underwent biopsy/re-resection at recurrence, 9 of 11 (82 %) had no evidence of EGFRvIII expression in the recurrent tumor [26]. These results suggest that the vaccine was effective in eradicating its target, but facilitated selection of a resistant tumor at recurrence.

To address the concern of limited efficacy with a single antigenic target, a new generation of multivalent peptide vaccines is now in clinical trials for GBM. The peptide vaccine SL-701 is a proprietary multivalent vaccine that has been tested for a mixed group of pediatric high-grade gliomas in a phase I trial with evidence of a positive immunologic response in 81 % of patients [29]. A phase I/II study is now enrolling adult patients with recurrent GBM (NCT02078648). The IMA950 platform contains a proprietary group of 11 synthetic HLA-A2 restricted tumor-associated peptides (TUMAPs) identified by screening a large number of GBM samples [30]. This multivalent peptide vaccine is being studied in patients with newly diagnosed GBM when given in combination with GM-CSF (NCT01222221). A phase I/II study of IMA950 in combination with Poly-ICLC is now recruiting patients as well (NCT01920191). Enrollment in this trial is still limited to HLA-A2 positive patients and it is unclear how many of the target peptides the average individual patient actually expresses.

2.2 Dendritic Cell Vaccines

In contrast to peptide vaccines that rely on endogenous APCs to uptake and display the peptide for T cell stimulation, DC vaccines control this crucial step by ex vivo manipulation. DC vaccines are generated after harvesting a patient's autologous DCs by plasmapheresis. Cells are stimulated ex vivo and antigenic peptides are introduced by pulsing them with DCs in culture. Activated DCs expressing the antigenic peptides on class I MHC are then reintroduced systemically, facilitating education of naïve T cells. This approach was used for the first cancer vaccine approved by the FDA, developed for the treatment of prostate cancer [16]. In comparison to peptide vaccines that can be given "off the shelf", this personalized vaccine approach is much more labor intensive and expensive. However, while peptide vaccines require predetermination of the antigenic target to synthesize the immune-stimulatory peptide, DCs can be pulsed with selected peptides or whole tumor lysate, allowing development of a unique, multivalent vaccine targeting the most highly expressed antigens in a particular patient's tumor.

A number of early phase clinical trials utilizing DC vaccine for GBM have been completed and reported (Table 1). The ICT-107 vaccine utilizes a panel of six HLA-A1/2 restricted peptides known to be highly expressed in glioma stem cells that are pulsed into autologous DCs for generation of the vaccine. In a small phase I study, the vaccine demonstrated highly hopeful results in 17 newly diagnosed GBM patients with a median PFS of 16.9 months and median OS of 38.4 months [31]. This led to a randomized, placebo-controlled phase IIb trial for newly diagnosed GBM (NCT01280552). Although not yet published, the results have been reported, demonstrating that the median OS in 81 vaccine treated patients was only 18.3 months with no significant differences in the treatment and placebo arms. Other DC vaccines with selected glioma-associated antigens have shown similar median OS of approximately 18 months in early phase trials with mixed high-grade gliomas [32].

Capitalizing on the advantages of the DC approach, a number of studies have utilized whole tumor lysate pulsed into DCs to develop a patient-specific multivalent vaccine. Single arm phase I/II trials utilizing this approach in mixed populations of newly diagnosed and recurrent GBM have demonstrated median PFS of 8–18 months with median OS of 18–34 months [33, 34]. It is difficult to assess efficacy in these small, single arm trials with mixed populations of newly diagnosed and recurrent GBM patients, as well as some anaplastic astrocytoma patients. These trials do, however, clearly demonstrate a robust immune response in the majority of patients in response to vaccination [33]. A number of other early phase trials of DC vaccine with more homogenous populations are currently ongoing (Table 1). In addition, a phase III, randomized, placebo-controlled trial of the DCVax-L vaccine, an autologous tumor lysate pulsed DC vaccine, is currently underway for newly diagnosed GBM patients (NCT00045968). The results of this trial are highly awaited and will be an important determinant of the viability of DC vaccines for the treatment of GBM.

2.3 Heat Shock Protein Vaccines

An alternative method to deliver antigenic peptides to APCs for presentation to naïve T cells is the use of heat shock proteins. HSPs are intracellular chaperones involved in trafficking peptides throughout an active cell. They are ubiquitously expressed in all cells, but particularly in cells under stress, such as neoplasms. Members of the HSP family, such as HSP 70 and 96, have specialized mechanisms to deliver antigenic peptides to APCs for presentation [35]. Peptides bound to HSP-96 in the extracellular environment can be internalized into endogenous DCs through the CD91 receptor, resulting in cleavage of the peptide and expression of the antigen on class I and II MHC [36]. By extracting HSP-96 with its associated peptides from whole tumor lysate, a personalized polyvalent vaccine can be generated. HSP vaccines are easier and more cost-effective to produce than DC vaccine, while maintaining the personalized polyvalent antigen expression not available with peptide vaccines.

A heat shock protein peptide complex-96 (HSPPC-96) vaccine has been developed and tested in newly diagnosed and recurrent GBM in phase I/II trials. In a phase I study, 11 of 12 vaccinated patients were found to have a significant peripheral immune response to intradermal vaccination [37]. In a phase II study for recurrent GBM in 41 patients, median PFS was 5 months and median OS was 10.5 months [38]. The phase II study for newly diagnosed GBM has not been published, but early results in 46 patients demonstrate a median PFS of 16 months and median OS of 23.3 months [39]. These single arm results are promising, but randomized, controlled phase II/III trials are necessary to assess the true clinical benefit. A phase IIb trial of the HSPPC-96 vaccine with bevacizumab versus bevacizumab alone for recurrent GBM is currently ongoing (NCT01814813).

3 Immune Modulators

While the results of early phase clinical trials for glioma vaccines demonstrate promising results, the survival benefit among highly selected patient populations is on the order of months, rather than years or decades. In most of these trials, a positive immune-stimulatory response to vaccination has been measured. So, why are not the benefits of immunotherapy greater? In general, cancer is known to be highly immunosuppressive. This is particularly true of gliomas. Multiple studies have demonstrated that patients with gliomas have reduced leukocyte counts and impaired leukocyte function, a phenomenon that worsens with the grade of the tumor [40–42]. The mechanisms of local immunoresistance and systemic immunosuppression are multifactorial, but a few key factors have been identified in GBM and other cancers.

3.1 Regulatory T Cells

Regulatory T cells (Tregs) are a subclass of $CD4^{+}$ T cells that exert an immunosuppressive effect on APCs and effector T cells through the production of immunosuppressive cytokines such as IL-10 and TGF-b [43]. Tregs (defined as $CD4^{+}$, $CD25^{+}$, $FoxP3^{+}$) are enriched in the blood and tumor of patients with GBM, establishing an immunosuppressive environment [44–46]. Soluble factors secreted from the tumor have been shown to recruit and expand Tregs, and therefore the degree of immunosuppression is proportional to the tumor burden [47]. Experimental depletion of Tregs in animal models of gliomas has been shown to improve survival [48]. Humanized monoclonal antibodies targeting the alpha subunit of the IL-2 receptor (CD25) are now available for clinical use. Although developed to modulate autoimmune diseases, these agents have been used in small pilot studies for GBM in combination with vaccine immunotherapy to deplete Tregs. When daclizumab was given to patients with newly diagnosed GBM in combination with an EGFRvIII peptide vaccine, a significant reduction in Tregs was demonstrated relative to saline-injected control patients [49]. Additionally, patients with decreased Tregs mounted a greater humoral response to vaccination, as had been previously shown in other studies [50]. A phase I study of basiliximab in combination with a DC vaccine is currently ongoing (NCT00626483).

3.2 CTLA-4

Normal activation of effector T cells involves binding of the specific T cell receptor to its antigenic target displayed on the MHC of an APC. Activation also requires binding of a cofactor (B7.1/B7.2) on the APC with its receptor (CD28) on the T cell. However, B7 can also bind to the CTLA-4 receptor on T cells resulting in the opposite effect, T cell inactivation [51]. The balance of binding to CD28 versus CTLA-4 determines the relative activity of systemic T cells. Inhibiting CTLA-4 can increase overall T cell reactivity and boost systemic immunity [4]. Inhibitors of CTLA-4, such as ipilimumab, have been shown to modulate the immune response to cancer in melanoma patients and can successfully improve survival when used as monotherapy or in combination with vaccines [52]. Although there is limited data on CTLA-4 expression in circulating T cells in GBM, the use of ipilumumab in GBM has been suggested and is part of a 3-arm trial of immunomodulators versus bevacizumab for recurrent GBM currently in a phase II trial (NCT02017717). Since Tregs are also known to express high levels of CTLA-4, CTLA-4 inhibitors, may function in part by modulating Treg activity as well [15].

3.3 PD-L1

T cell activity is also modulated by the immune checkpoint regulator programmed death ligand 1 (PD-L1), also known as B7 homologue 1 (B7-H1). PD-L1 is normally expressed on a variety of immune cells and can bind to its receptor, programmed death 1 (PD-1), on T cells, inducing T cell apoptosis or anergy. It is now well recognized that expression of PD-L1 on the surface of cancer cells results in immunoresistance in the tumor microenvironment [53]. Inhibitors of PD-L1 and the PD-1 receptor have been tested in early phase clinical trials for a variety of advanced solid organ tumors, demonstrating significant tumor regression in a small subset of patients [54, 55]. In GBM, expression of PD-L1 on the surface of tumor cells has been linked to loss of PTEN and overactivation of the PI3(k)-Akt pathway [56]. Tumor expression of PD-L1 contributes to local immunoresistence in GBM in a subset of patients with elevated expression [57]. However, most GBM patients are known to be systemically immunosuppressed with T cell dysfunction in circulation [41]. Recently, it has been identified that GBM patients also have increased PD-L1 expression on circulating monocytes and tumor-infiltrating macrophages, leading to a tumor-independent mechanism of immunosuppression [58]. Expression of PD-L1 on circulating monocytes has been shown to correlate with significantly worsened survival in patients who received the HSPPC-96 vaccine for newly diagnosed GBM [39]. A phase II trial of nivolumab, a PD-1 inhibitor, is currently ongoing for patients with recurrent GBM (NCT02017717).

4 Discussion

Immunotherapy for the treatment of cancer offers the possibility of a highly specific, minimally toxic alternative to chemotherapy, with the benefit of sustained efficacy provided that immunologic memory is induced. While immunotherapy comes in many forms, immune recognition of tumor-specific antigens by endogenous exposure or exogenous introduction of antigenic peptides is necessary for efficacy. Due to the lack of systemic metastasis by gliomas and their immune-privileged space behind the BBB, it is often believed that active vaccination is necessary to mount an immune response to gliomas. Nearly all active immunotherapy trials of GBM to date have been vaccine trials with or without an immune stimulating adjuvant. As presented, the results of a number of phase I/II trials for glioma vaccines demonstrate moderate improvement in survival as compared to historical controls. Dramatic effects of glioma vaccines are limited by the challenge of immunosuppression and local tumor immunoresistance. The mechanisms underlying the immunosuppression, including expansion of Tregs, CTLA-4 expression, and PD-L1/PD-1 interaction, have just recently been fully elucidated. Targeting these factors with immune modulating therapy has been successful in other cancers, but those other tumors are known to metastasize hematogenously and to be highly immunoreactive at baseline. Although a trial of PD-1 inhibition with and without CTLA-4 inhibition is currently ongoing for recurrent GBM, it is not clear that immune checkpoint modulation alone is sufficient to mount a robust immune response in GBM. More likely, a combined approach of active vaccination with immunomodulation to boost the response will be the most effective therapy for gliomas. Such combined therapy is not currently part of any active clinical trial, but is being planned for a number of vaccine approaches. Immunotherapy for cancer, and particularly for gliomas, is still in its early stages, but as our understanding of the critical factors in cancer immunology matures, immunotherapy will likely play a larger part in the treatment of malignant gliomas.

References

1. Dunn GP, Old LJ, Schreiber RD (2004) The immunobiology of cancer immunosurveillance and immunoediting. Immunity 21:137–148. doi:10.1016/j.immuni.2004.07.017, pii: S1074761304002092
2. Schreiber RD, Old LJ, Smyth MJ (2011) Cancer immunoediting: integrating immunity's roles in cancer suppression and promotion. Science 331:1565–1570. doi:10.1126/science.1203486, pii:331/6024/1565
3. Grulich AE, van Leeuwen MT, Falster MO, Vajdic CM (2007) Incidence of cancers in people with HIV/AIDS compared with immunosuppressed transplant recipients: a meta-analysis. Lancet 370: 59–67. doi:10.1016/S0140-6736(07)61050-2, pii:S0140-6736(07)61050-2
4. Raval RR, Sharabi AB, Walker AJ, Drake CG, Sharma P (2014) Tumor immunology and cancer immunotherapy: summary of the 2013 SITC primer. J Immunother Cancer 2:14. doi:10.1186/2051-1426-2-14, pii:2051-1426-2-14
5. Slamon DJ, Leyland-Jones B, Shak S et al (2001) Use of chemotherapy plus a monoclonal antibody against HER2 for metastatic breast cancer that overexpresses HER2. N Engl J Med 344:783–792. doi:10.1056/NEJM200103153441101
6. Peinert S, Kershaw MH, Prince HM (2009) Chimeric T cells for adoptive immunotherapy of cancer: using what have we learned to plan for the future. Immunotherapy 1:905–912. doi: 10.2217/imt.09.69
7. Mellman I, Coukos G, Dranoff G (2011) Cancer immunotherapy comes of age. Nature 480:480–489. doi:10.1038/nature10673, pii:nature10673
8. Mukherji B, Chakraborty NG, Sivanandham M (1990) T-cell clones that react against autologous human tumors. Immunol Rev 116:33–62
9. Berke G (1995) The CTL's kiss of death. Cell 81(1):9–12. doi:10.1016/0092-8674(95)90365-8,pii:0092-8674(95)90365-8
10. Grimm EA, Owen-Schaub L (1991) The IL-2 mediated amplification of cellular cytotoxicity. J Cell Biochem 45:335–339. doi:10.1002/jcb.240450405

11. McDermott DF, Regan MM, Clark JI et al (2005) Randomized phase III trial of high-dose interleukin-2 versus subcutaneous interleukin-2 and interferon in patients with metastatic renal cell carcinoma. J Clin Oncol 23:133–141. doi:10.1200/JCO.2005.03.206, pii:23/1/133
12. Sparano JA, Fisher RI, Sunderland M et al (1993) Randomized phase III trial of treatment with high-dose interleukin-2 either alone or in combination with interferon alfa-2a in patients with advanced melanoma. J Clin Oncol 11:1969–1977
13. Lu H (2014) TLR agonists for cancer immunotherapy: tipping the balance between the immune stimulatory and inhibitory effects. Front Immunol 5:83. doi:10.3389/fimmu.2014.00083
14. Pardoll DM (2012) The blockade of immune checkpoints in cancer immunotherapy. Nat Rev Cancer 12:252–264. doi:10.1038/nrc3239, pii:nrc3239
15. Curran MA, Montalvo W, Yagita H, Allison JP (2010) PD-1 and CTLA-4 combination blockade expands infiltrating T cells and reduces regulatory T and myeloid cells within B16 melanoma tumors. Proc Natl Acad Sci USA 107:4275–4280. doi:10.1073/pnas.0915174107, pii:0915174107
16. Kantoff PW, Higano CS, Shore ND et al (2010) Sipuleucel-T immunotherapy for castration-resistant prostate cancer. N Engl J Med 363:411–422. doi:10.1056/NEJMoa1001294
17. Dunn GP, Old LJ, Schreiber RD (2004) The three Es of cancer immunoediting. Annu Rev Immunol 22:329–360. doi:10.1146/annurev.immunol.22.012703.104803
18. Carpentier PA, Begolka WS, Olson JK, Elhofy A, Karpus WJ, Miller SD (2005) Differential activation of astrocytes by innate and adaptive immune stimuli. Glia 49:360–374. doi:10.1002/glia.20117
19. Dong Y, Benveniste EN (2001) Immune function of astrocytes. Glia 36(2):180–190. doi:10.1002/glia.1107,pii:glia.1107
20. Pachter JS, de Vries HE, Fabry Z (2003) The blood-brain barrier and its role in immune privilege in the central nervous system. J Neuropathol Exp Neurol 62:593–604
21. Giometto B, Bozza F, Faresin F, Alessio L, Mingrino S, Tavolato B (1996) Immune infiltrates and cytokines in gliomas. Acta Neurochir (Wien) 138:50–56
22. Parney IF, Waldron JS, Parsa AT (2009) Flow cytometry and in vitro analysis of human glioma-associated macrophages. Laboratory investigation. J Neurosurg 110:572–582. doi:10.3171/2008.7.JNS08475, pii:10.3171/2008.7.JNS08475
23. Hatanpaa KJ, Burma S, Zhao D, Habib AA (2010) Epidermal growth factor receptor in glioma: signal transduction, neuropathology, imaging, and radioresistance. Neoplasia 12:675–684
24. Gan HK, Kaye AH, Luwor RB (2009) The EGFRvIII variant in glioblastoma multiforme. J Clin Neurosci 16:748–754. doi:10.1016/j.jocn.2008.12.005, pii:S0967-5868(09)00046-0
25. Heimberger AB, Sampson JH (2009) The PEPvIII-KLH (CDX-110) vaccine in glioblastoma multiforme patients. Expert Opin Biol Ther 9:1087–1098. doi:10.1517/14712590903124346
26. Sampson JH, Heimberger AB, Archer GE et al (2010) Immunologic escape after prolonged progression-free survival with epidermal growth factor receptor variant III peptide vaccination in patients with newly diagnosed glioblastoma. J Clin Oncol 28:4722–4729. doi:10.1200/JCO.2010.28.6963, pii:JCO.2010.28.6963
27. Izumoto S, Tsuboi A, Oka Y et al (2008) Phase II clinical trial of Wilms tumor 1 peptide vaccination for patients with recurrent glioblastoma multiforme. J Neurosurg 108:963–971. doi:10.3171/JNS/2008/108/5/0963
28. Sottoriva A, Spiteri I, Piccirillo SG, Touloumis A, Collins VP, Marioni JC, Curtis C, Watts C, Tavare S (2013) Intratumor heterogeneity in human glioblastoma reflects cancer evolutionary dynamics. Proc Natl Acad Sci USA 110:4009–4014. doi:10.1073/pnas.1219747110, pii:1219747110
29. Pollack IF, Jakacki RI, Butterfield LH et al (2014) Antigen-specific immune responses and clinical outcome after vaccination with glioma-associated antigen peptides and polyinosinic-polycytidylic acid stabilized by lysine and carboxymethylcellulose in children with newly diagnosed malignant brainstem and nonbrainstem gliomas. J Clin Oncol. doi:10.1200/JCO.2013.54.0526, pii:JCO.2013.54.0526

30. Dutoit V, Herold-Mende C, Hilf N et al (2012) Exploiting the glioblastoma peptidome to discover novel tumour-associated antigens for immunotherapy. Brain 135:1042–1054. doi:10.1093/brain/aws042, pii:aws042
31. Phuphanich S, Wheeler CJ, Rudnick JD et al (2013) Phase I trial of a multi-epitope-pulsed dendritic cell vaccine for patients with newly diagnosed glioblastoma. Cancer Immunol Immunother 62:125–135. doi:10.1007/s00262-012-1319-0
32. Prins RM, Wang X, Soto H et al (2013) Comparison of glioma-associated antigen peptide-loaded versus autologous tumor lysate-loaded dendritic cell vaccination in malignant glioma patients. J Immunother 36:152–157. doi:10.1097/CJI.0b013e3182811ae4
33. Liau LM, Prins RM, Kiertscher SM et al (2005) Dendritic cell vaccination in glioblastoma patients induces systemic and intracranial T-cell responses modulated by the local central nervous system tumor microenvironment. Clin Cancer Res 11:5515–5525. doi:10.1158/1078-0432.CCR-05-0464, pii:11/15/5515
34. Wheeler CJ, Black KL, Liu G et al. (2008) Vaccination elicits correlated immune and clinical responses in glioblastoma multiforme patients. Cancer Res 68:5955–5964. doi:10.1158/0008-5472.CAN-07-5973, pii:68/14/5955
35. Srivastava PK, Callahan MK, Mauri MM (2009) Treating human cancers with heat shock protein-peptide complexes: the road ahead. Expert Opin Biol Ther 9:179–186. doi:10.1517/14712590802633918
36. Binder RJ, Srivastava PK (2004) Essential role of CD91 in re-presentation of gp96-chaperoned peptides. Proc Natl Acad Sci USA 101:6128–6133. doi:10.1073/pnas.0308180101, pii:0308180101
37. Crane CA, Han SJ, Ahn B et al (2013) Individual patient-specific immunity against high-grade glioma after vaccination with autologous tumor derived peptides bound to the 96 KD chaperone protein. Clin Cancer Res 19:205–214. doi:10.1158/1078-0432.CCR-11-3358, pii:1078-0432.CCR-11-3358
38. Bloch O, Crane CA, Fuks Y et al (2014) Heat-shock protein peptide complex-96 vaccination for recurrent glioblastoma: a phase II, single-arm trial. Neuro Oncol 16:274–279. doi:10.1093/neuonc/not203, pii:not203
39. Bloch O, Kaur R, Aghi MK, McDermott MW, Berger MS, Parsa AT (2013) Glioma-induced immunosuppression shortens progression-free survival in a trial of immunotherapy for glioblastoma. In: American association of neurological surgeons annual meeting, New Orleans, LA
40. Brooks WH, Netsky MG, Normansell DE, Horwitz DA (1972) Depressed cell-mediated immunity in patients with primary intracranial tumors. Characterization of a humoral immunosuppressive factor. J Exp Med 136:1631–1647
41. Elliott LH, Brooks WH, Roszman TL (1984) Cytokinetic basis for the impaired activation of lymphocytes from patients with primary intracranial tumors. J Immunol 132:1208–1215
42. Gousias K, Markou M, Arzoglou V, Voulgaris S, Vartholomatos G, Kostoula A, Voulgari P, Polyzoidis K, Kyritsis AP (2010) Frequent abnormalities of the immune system in gliomas and correlation with the WHO grading system of malignancy. J Neuroimmunol 226: 36–42. doi:10.1016/j.jneuroim.2010.05.027, pii:S0165-5728(10)00211-0
43. Facciabene A, Motz GT, Coukos G (2012) T-regulatory cells: key players in tumor immune escape and angiogenesis. Cancer Res 72:2162–2171. doi:10.1158/0008-5472.CAN-11-3687, pii:72/9/2162
44. Fecci PE, Mitchell DA, Whitesides JF et al (2006) Increased regulatory T-cell fraction amidst a diminished CD4 compartment explains cellular immune defects in patients with malignant glioma. Cancer Res 66:3294–3302. doi:10.1158/0008-5472.CAN-05-3773, pii:66/6/3294
45. Heimberger AB, Abou-Ghazal M, Reina-Ortiz C, Yang DS, Sun W, Qiao W, Hiraoka N, Fuller GN (2008) Incidence and prognostic impact of FoxP3+ regulatory T cells in human gliomas. Clin Cancer Res 14:5166–5172. doi:10.1158/1078-0432.CCR-08-0320, pii:14/16/5166
46. Learn CA, Fecci PE, Schmittling RJ et al. (2006) Profiling of CD4+, CD8+, and CD4+ CD25+ CD45RO+ FoxP3+ T cells in patients with malignant glioma reveals differential expression of the immunologic transcriptome compared with T cells from healthy volunteers. Clin Cancer Res 12:7306–7315. doi:10.1158/1078-0432.CCR-06-1727, pii:12/24/7306

47. Crane CA, Ahn BJ, Han SJ, Parsa AT (2012) Soluble factors secreted by glioblastoma cell lines facilitate recruitment, survival, and expansion of regulatory T cells: implications for immunotherapy. Neuro Oncol 14:584–595. doi:10.1093/neuonc/nos014, pii:nos014
48. El Andaloussi A, Han Y, Lesniak MS (2006) Prolongation of survival following depletion of CD4+ CD25+ regulatory T cells in mice with experimental brain tumors. J Neurosurg 105:430–437. doi:10.3171/jns.2006.105.3.430
49. Sampson JH, Schmittling RJ, Archer GE et al (2012) A pilot study of IL-2Ralpha blockade during lymphopenia depletes regulatory T-cells and correlates with enhanced immunity in patients with glioblastoma. PLoS One 7:e31046. doi:10.1371/journal.pone.0031046, pii:PONE-D-11-20574
50. Fong B, Jin R, Wang X, Safaee M, Lisiero DN, Yang I, Li G, Liau LM, Prins RM (2012) Monitoring of regulatory T cell frequencies and expression of CTLA-4 on T cells, before and after DC vaccination, can predict survival in GBM patients. PLoS One 7:e32614. doi:10.1371/journal.pone.0032614, pii:PONE-D-11-22564
51. Ceeraz S, Nowak EC, Noelle RJ (2013) B7 family checkpoint regulators in immune regulation and disease. Trends Immunol 34:556–563. doi:10.1016/j.it.2013.07.003, pii:S1471-4906(13)00110-5
52. Hodi FS, O'Day SJ, McDermott DF et al (2010) Improved survival with ipilimumab in patients with metastatic melanoma. N Engl J Med 363:711–723. doi:10.1056/NEJMoa1003466, pii:NEJMoa1003466
53. Dong H, Strome SE, Salomao DR et al (2002) Tumor-associated B7-H1 promotes T-cell apoptosis: a potential mechanism of immune evasion. Nat Med 8:793–800. doi:10.1038/nm730, pii:nm730
54. Brahmer JR, Tykodi SS, Chow LQ et al (2012) Safety and activity of anti-PD-L1 antibody in patients with advanced cancer. N Engl J Med 366:2455–2465. doi:10.1056/NEJMoa1200694
55. Topalian SL, Hodi FS, Brahmer JR et al (2012) Safety, activity, and immune correlates of anti-PD-1 antibody in cancer. N Engl J Med 366:2443–2454. doi:10.1056/NEJMoa1200690
56. Parsa AT, Waldron JS, Panner A et al (2007) Loss of tumor suppressor PTEN function increases B7-H1 expression and immunoresistance in glioma. Nat Med 13:84–88. doi:10.1038/nm1517, pii:nm1517
57. Wintterle S, Schreiner B, Mitsdoerffer M, Schneider D, Chen L, Meyermann R, Weller M, Wiendl H (2003) Expression of the B7-related molecule B7-H1 by glioma cells: a potential mechanism of immune paralysis. Cancer Res 63:7462–7467
58. Bloch O, Crane CA, Kaur R, Safaee M, Rutkowski MJ, Parsa AT (2013) Gliomas promote immunosuppression through induction of B7-H1 expression in tumor-associated macrophages. Clin Cancer Res 19:3165–3175. doi:10.1158/1078-0432.CCR-12-3314, pii:1078-0432.CCR-12-3314
59. Vik-Mo EO, Nyakas M, Mikkelsen BV, Moe MC, Due-Tønnesen P, Suso EM, Sæbøe-Larssen S, Sandberg C, Brinchmann JE, Helseth E, Rasmussen AM, Lote K, Aamdal S, Gaudernack G, Kvalheim G, Langmoen IA (2013) Therapeutic vaccination against autologous cancer stem cells with mRNA-transfected dendritic cells in patients with glioblastoma. Cancer ImmunolImmunother 62(9):1499–1509. doi:10.1007/s00262-013-1453-3
60. Fadul CE, Fisher JL, Hampton TH, Lallana EC, Li Z, Gui J, Szczepiorkowski ZM, Tosteson TD, Rhodes CH, Wishart HA, Lewis LD, Ernstoff MS (2011) Immune response in patients with newly diagnosed glioblastomamultiforme treated with intranodal autologous tumor lysate-dendritic cell vaccination after radiation chemotherapy. J Immunother 34(4):382–389. doi:10.1097/CJI.0b013e318215e300
61. Wen PY, Reardon DA, Phuphanich S, Aiken R, Landolfi JC, Curry WT, Zhu JJ, Glantz MJ, Peereboom DM, Markert J, LaRocca RV, O'Rourke D, Fink KL, Kim LJ, Gruber ML, Lesser GJ, Pan E, Kesari S, Hawkins ES, Yu J (2014) A randomized, double-blind, placebo-controlled phase 2 trial of dendritic cell (DC) vaccination with ICT-107 in newly diagnosed glioblastoma (GBM) patients. J Clin Oncol 32:5s (suppl; abstract number 2005)

62. Lai R, Recht LD, Reardon DA, Paleologos N, Groves MD, Rosenfeld MR, Meech S, Davis TA, Pavlov D, Sampson JH (2010) Interim data for ACT III: phase II trial of PF-04948568 (CDX-110) in combination with temozolomide (TMZ) in patients with glioblastoma (GBM). J Clin Oncol 28:15s (suppl; abstract number 2014)

Glioblastoma in the Elderly

Marc C. Chamberlain

Abstract There is no generally agreed upon standard of care treatment for elderly patients (age ≥70 years) with glioblastoma (GBM). Treatment options range from supportive care only, radiation therapy (RT) only (most often given in a shortened hypofractionated schedule), temozolomide (TMZ) chemotherapy only, and the combination RT + TMZ, followed by post-RT TMZ as is the current standard of care for younger good performance patients with newly diagnosed GBM.

Keyword Glioblastoma · Elderly patients · Hypofractionated radiotherapy · Temozolomide

Contents

1 Introduction

The recently published randomized European Organization for Research and Treatment of Cancer and National Cancer Institute of Canada trial (EORTC/NCIC) substantially altered the algorithm for initial treatment of glioblastoma (GBM) [1]. This study of 573 patients demonstrated a statistically significant benefit (as determined by a 2.5 month improvement in median overall survival [mOS] when

M.C. Chamberlain (✉)
Department of Neurology and Neurological Surgery, University of Washington/Fred Hutchison Cancer Research Center, Seattle Cancer Care Alliance, 825 Eastlake Ave East MS G4940, Box 19023, Seattle, WA 98109, USA
e-mail: chambemc@uw.edu

J. Raizer and A. Parsa (eds.), *Current Understanding and Treatment of Gliomas*, Cancer Treatment and Research 163, DOI 10.1007/978-3-319-12048-5_10

Table 1 Radiation therapy oncology group recursive partitioning classification system

Class^	Median overall survival (months)	2-year survival (%)
1	58	76
2	37	68
3*	18	35
4*	11	15
5*	9	6
6*	4.5	4

Legend ^Class defined by age, performance status, histology, neurological function and duration of symptoms
*Glioblastoma containing classes

Table 2 Hazard ration by age group in the EORTC/NCIC trial

Age, years (number of patients)	Hazard ratio	*P* value
<50 (171)	0.5	0.001
50–60 (220)	0.63	<0.05
61–65 (*)	0.72	0.096
66–71 (*)	0.8	0.34

*Age 61–71 years total number 173

compared to RT only) for chemotherapy (temozolomide [TMZ] given concurrently with radiotherapy [RT], followed by 6 monthly cycles of TMZ) in the initial treatment of good performance patients (Eastern Cooperative Oncology Group [ECOG] performance 0–2) with GBM. Notably, however, the study design excluded patients ≥70 years of age, a group of patients constituting >25 % of all newly diagnosed GBM [2–4]. Patients over the age of 70 years are most commonly defined as the elderly, though some definitions include patients aged 65 years and older. In a recent analysis of the EORTC/NCIC trial study, population stratified by the Radiation Therapy Oncology Group Recursive Partitioning Analysis (RTOG RPA) Class, benefit of RT + concomitant and adjuvant TMZ (RT + TMZ) was seen only in Class 3 and 4 patients (Table 1) [5]. In that more than 50 % of all elderly patients with GBM are characterized as RTOG RPA Class 5 or 6, RT only until recently was the standard treatment notwithstanding modest survival results [6, 7]. In that patients over the age of 70 years were not included in the landmark EORTC/NCIC trial, the question of the applicability of this regimen to patients over the age of 70 remains controversial. The utility of the EORTC/NCIC regimen of radiotherapy and concurrent and adjuvant TMZ was never well-defined for older patients with GBM and as seen in unpublished data from the EORTC Data Center in Table 2 (personal communication from Dr. James Perry), little benefit of this treatment strategy is apparent in patients >65 years of age. Currently, there are several treatment approaches to this demographically enlarging elderly patient population (Table 3). The diversity of treatments reflects both the limited prospective clinical trials in this patient population as well as a belief that standard of care (SOC) RT + TMZ followed by TMZ is of benefit, particularly in physiologically fit elderly patients with good performance [8–11].

Table 3 Treatment options for newly diagnosed elderly patients with glioblastoma

Treatment	Treatment parameters	Indication	Evidence
Radiation therapy only	40 Gy in 15 fractions	If MGMT methylation status not known or unmethylated	Evidenced-based
Temozolomide monotherapy	150–200 mg/m2/day x5 days every 4 weeks	If *MGMT* promoter methylation is present	Evidenced-based
Best supportive care		Impaired performance status unable to care for oneself	Not evidenced-based
Combination therapy	Standard protocol of RT (60 Gy in 30 fractions) with concurrent TMZ followed by 6 cycles of postradiotherapy TMZ	Patients with good performance status (KPS > 60)	Not evidenced-based
Clinical trial	Standard of care (RT + TMZ followed by TMZ) with an investigational agent	Patients with a good performance status (KPS > 60) and having undergone tumor resection (for tissue molecular correlates)	Investigational therapy

Legend MGMT Methylguanine-methytransferase, *KPS* Karnofsky performance status, *RT* Radiotherapy, *TMZ* Temozolomide, *Gy* Gray

Age is recognized as the most important prognostic factor for survival in GBM and survival declines after age 50 (a primary node point identified in the RTOG RPA classification system) [12]. Furthermore, there is a near linear decline in survival in patients with GBM greater than 50 years of age [3–5, 8]. Population-based studies of patients with newly diagnosed GBM show a mOS of 6 months in elderly patients, which is significantly lower than in younger patients [3, 5–7].

In addition to age, performance status (PS) is considered the second most relevant prognostic factor for survival in patients with GBM. Similar to patients >70 years of age, patients with markedly diminished or impoverished PS defined as an ECOG PS > 2 or a KPS < 60 have a mOS of 6 months or less. Because performance is so strongly correlated with survival, all current and most recent trials of newly diagnosed GBM only include patients with good performance status as defined by an ECOG performance score of 0–2 or a Karnofsky performance status of >60. These levels of performance imply independence in activities of daily living.

Two other relevant prognostic factors that are germane to elderly patients with GBM include tumor content of the DNA damage repair enzyme, methylguanine methyltransferase (*MGMT*), and the tumor mutational status of the isocitrate dehydrogenase 1 (*IDH1*) enzyme [13–17]. Patients with low tumor content of *MGMT*, a result of epigenetic silencing of the *MGMT* gene by promoter methylation, results in tumors with increased susceptibility to alkylator chemotherapy-induced injury. In elderly patients, the incidence of *MGMT* promoter methylated tumors is either higher (50 % as assessed by the German Glioma Network) or similar to that seen in younger adult patients (30–40 %) suggesting either no age dependence of *MGMT* methylation or possibly an increase with age [18–20]. Regardless *MGMT* promoter methylation status does not appear to adversely influence outcome in elderly patients with GBM. By contrast, *IDH1* mutated gliomas currently defined as so-called secondary GBM, that is a GBM that arises from a lower grade glioma, have been demonstrated to have a more favorable outcome irrespective of treatment than the far more common (>90 %) primary GBM that arise de novo. The incidence of secondary GBM, however, decreases with age and, in contrast to *MGMT* promoter methylation, *IDH1* mutations are age dependent and only rarely manifest in GBM of elderly patients (<2 %) [21]. The rarity of *IDH1* mutated secondary GBM in the elderly may in part contribute to the above-mentioned poor overall survival.

Germane to treatment of elderly patients with GBM, geriatric oncologists recognize three categories of elderly patients based upon performance status, medical comorbidities, and age [22]. Frail elderly patients are defined by age >85 years (a category considered the oldest old), dependence in one or more activities of daily living, one or more medical comorbidities and one or more geriatric syndromes (defined as delirium, dementia, depression, osteoporosis, incontinence, falls, or failure to thrive). Physiologically, young elderly patients (as assessed by a geriatric scale) are defined by age <80 years, independence in activities of living, minimal to no medical comorbidities and no geriatric syndrome. The majority of clinical trials discussed below primarily relate to this category of elderly patient. The last category of elderly patients is those with a compromised PS that are dependent upon others in most or all activities of daily living. This category of elderly as well as younger patients with compromised PS is nearly always excluded from clinical trials due very limited survival.

2 Treatment

Several population-based studies document elderly patients with GBM receive less therapy than younger patients [3, 6, 7, 11, 23–25]. Of note the majority of published data on patterns of care in the elderly with GBM are derived before TMZ became available.

A SEER database analysis of 4,137 patients >65 years of age who were treated between 1994 and 2002 demonstrated that advancing age was associated with decreased use of resection, RT and chemotherapy, and with a diminished survival (mOS 4 months) [10]. A second SEER database analysis on 2,836 patients over the age of 70 showed that 86 % of patients received some form of treatment, but that only 46 % of patients underwent both surgery and RT [11]. In addition, another study reported that the rate of treatment with supportive care only increased with age [6]. A reason posited for diminished care in the elderly was the concern for increased toxicity from treatment with increasing age, patient preference, and the treating physician's perceived treatment nihilism.

Until recently, there was a paucity of randomized clinical trials for the elderly GBM patient population and consequently the most appropriate treatment for this large cohort of patients with newly diagnosed GBM was ill-defined and controversial (Table 4). Two previous randomized studies in elderly GBM patients demonstrated that involved field fractionated radiotherapy (RT50: 50 Gy in 28 fractions) is superior to supportive care only (median survival 7 vs. 4 months) and that conventional fractioned RT (sdRT; total dose 60 Gy in 30 fractions) is comparable to hypofractionated RT (hypoRT; 40 Gy in 15 fractions) [6, 7]. These trials provided evidence to commend in elderly patients with GBM and deemed candidates for treatment that hypoRT should serve as the standard of care for this subpopulation. Several subsequent retrospective studies suggested an alternative treatment that is standard dose TMZ (sdTMZ) with deferred RT, however, these studies constituted low level of evidence [26, 27].

A recent prospective randomized German study (NOA-08 study) compared up-front TMZ in a dose-dense regimen (ddTMZ is given at 100 mg/m^2/day for 7 consecutive days every 14 days) versus conventional fractioned RT (RT60: 60 Gy in 30 fractions) to elderly patients with high-grade glioma [HGG] (defined as age >65 years, KPS ≥ 60, and tumor histology GBM or anaplastic astrocytoma) {median survival 8.6 months vs. 9.6 months} [18]. The primary endpoint was overall survival and the trial design was that of a noninferiority endpoint. Median overall survival in the ddTMZ arm was 8.6 months versus 9.6 months in the sdRT arm demonstrating noninferiority between these two treatment regimens. As a consequence of this study, an evidence-based conclusion would be that TMZ may be administered as an alternative to elderly patients with GBM as opposed to sdRT. What remains unclear notwithstanding the above-mentioned three randomized trials is how to treat elderly patients with GBM that have an impoverished performance, a not uncommon situation that accounted in part for the reduced number of patients enrolled in the NOA-08 trial. Of 584 patients screened for NOA-08, only 373 patients were ultimately treated per protocol, the 209 patients [36 %] deemed ineligible were primarily due to poor PS. In addition, whether the use of ddTMZ as used in the NOA-08 trial is superior compared to the standard 5-day TMZ regimen (sdTMZ) is unclear. The recently completed Radiation Therapy Oncology Group study, RTOG 0525 in patients with newly diagnosed GBM demonstrated no survival benefit to post-RT ddTMZ [19]. Further, the recently completed Medical Research Council trial of chemotherapy for chemotherapy naïve HGG in first relapse after treatment with surgery and RT showed no benefit to ddTMZ compared to sdTMZ [28]. Dose dense TMZ as acknowledged by the NOA-08 authors is more toxic and costly and likely no more efficacious compared to sdTMZ.

The very recently published Nordic randomized trial (342 patients enrolled, 291 randomized) that compared sdTMZ to sdRT to hypoRT (30 Gy in 10 fractions) in elderly GBM patients (defined as age >60 years and KPS ≥ 50) suggests sdTMZ is equivalent with respect to survival when compared to the hypoRT and superior to sdRT (60 Gy in 30 fractions) treatment arm [median survival 8.3 vs. 7.5 vs. 6 months] [29]. Based upon this prospective study, it would appear treatment with

Table 4 Clinical trials in elderly glioblastoma

Trial (Reference)	Age (years)	Number	Treatment							Median overall survival (months)
			RT60	RT50	RT40	RT34	RT + TMZ	TMZ	BSC	
EORTC/NCIC [1]	60–70	173	x				x			10.9/11.8
NCIC [7]	>70	95	x		x					6.1/5.6
French [6]	>70	81		x					x	6.6/3.5
NOA-08 [18]	>65	412	x					x		9.6/8.6
Nordic [29]	60–69	100	x			x		x		7.5/7.0/7.9
	>70	191	x			x		x		5.2/7.1/9.0
ANOCEF [30]	>70 + Low PS							x		6.0
ANOCEF [31]	>70 + Low PS							x + Bev		6.0

Legend EORTC/NCIC European Organization for Research and Treatment of Cancer/National Cancer Institute, Canada, *NCIC* National Cancer Institute, Canada, *RT#* Radiotherapy total dose, *RT + TMZ* Radiotherapy plus concurrent and adjuvant temozolomide, *TMZ* Temozolomide, *BSC* Best standard of care, *Bev* Bevacizumab, *PS* Performance status either sdTMZ or hypoRT is equivalent for elderly GBM patients and importantly evidenced-based.

In a single arm multi-institutional Phase II study of 70 patients by the French consortium ANOCEF (Association de Neuro-Oncologie d'Expression Française) in patients with GBM, age >70 years, 90 % biopsy only and KPS < 70, sdTMZ only treatment resulted in a median overall survival of 6 months conferring further evidence of chemotherapy only for newly diagnosed elderly GBM is a valid treatment [30]. Very recently, a second French ANOCEF trial in newly diagnosed elderly patients with GBM assessed the benefit of adding bevacizumab to sdTMZ and when compared to the above-mentioned ANOCEF trial found no benefit to the up-front use of bevacizumab in combination with sdTMZ compared to sdTMZ only [31]. This ANOCEF study appears to recapitulate the large RTOG 0825 and European AVAglio trials that compared SOC RT + TMZ with or with bevacizumab in young good PS patients with newly diagnosed GBM and demonstrated no overall survival advantage for the up-front use of bevacizumab [32, 33].

In a retrospective series of 233 elderly patients with GBM (median age 74 years), the German Glioma Network concluded *MGMT* promoter methylation increases with increasing age, *MGMT* promoter methylation is prognostic for mOS but not for progression free survival (PFS), *MGMT* promoter methylated tumors have improved outcome when treated with alkylator chemotherapy versus RT and *MGMT* promoter unmethylated tumors have improved outcome when treated with RT versus chemotherapy [20]. Additionally, this large series assessed *MGMT* promoter methylation by two techniques; the commercially available and most frequently used methylation specific polymerase chain reaction (MSP) and by pyrosequencing. Pyrosequencing with >25 % *MGMT* methylated alleles (50 % all MSP positive tumors) better defined the cohort of patients most likely to respond to alkylator chemotherapy versus RT. Lastly, this study suggested that combined therapy (RT + TMZ) might be superior to TMZ only in the *MGMT* methylated group of tumors, whereas there was no added benefit of combination therapy over RT only in the *MGMT* unmethylated group of tumors. This latter point recapitulates results of the EORTC/NCIC trial discussed below.

A commonly recommended and frequently utilized treatment for elderly patients with GBM is the EORTC/NCIC regimen of TMZ-based chemoradiotherapy followed by 6-months of post-RT sdTMZ, a treatment that is established as the standard of care for patients <71 years of age and with a KPS ≥ 70 [1, 34–41]. Two recent randomized Phase III RTOG trials, 0525 mentioned above and 0825, a comparison of the EORTC/NCIC regimen with or without bevacizumab in newly diagnosed high PS patients with GBM undergoing resective surgery, have not provided any survival data on specific age cohorts [19, 32]. Consequently, it is uncertain if the RT + TMZ followed by post-RT sdTMZ regimen offers any benefit in elderly GMB patients, defined as patients >70 years and perhaps as young as >65 years of age, as compared to sdTMZ only or hypoRT.

In a subset analysis of the EORTC/NCIC trial, promoter methylation of the MGMT conferred a survival benefit suggesting both prognostic and predictive value of the MGMT promoter methylation status [13]. Importantly, this was confirmed prospectively in the RTOG 0525 trial [19]. Both trials suggested approximately 30 % of all newly diagnosed GBM are MGMT methylated and it is these patients which appear to gain benefit from the inclusion of TMZ. By contrast, the role of TMZ in the nonmethylated group is uncertain and lacking alternative therapies, both methylated and unmethylated GB patients continue to be treated with RT + TMZ regimen outside of clinical trials [3, 21, 22]. The German NOA-08 study ascertained MGMT methylation in a subset of patients (35 %) and determined that ddTMZ conferred a benefit with respect to event-free survival (statistically significant) and overall survival (trend only) compared to sdRT only (median survival 8.4 vs. 4.6 months) suggesting MGMT determination may be relevant for treatment decisions in elderly patients with GBM [18]. Similarly, the Nordic trial assessed MGMT status in 75 % of all patients and demonstrated a survival benefit in patients with MGMT methylated promoter when treated with sdTMZ as compared to unmethylated MGMT (median survival 9.7 vs. 6.8 months) [29]. MGMT promoter status (methylated or unmethylated) did not affect survival in patients treated with either RT treatment arm [28]. This conclusion is similar to that of the EORTC/NCIC trial and despite which patients with newly diagnosed GBM continue to be treated outside of clinical trials with RT + TMZ followed by post-RT sdTMZ [13]. It is unlikely another trial of newly diagnosed GBM will be conducted comparing RT to RT + TMZ that is powered sufficiently to conclusively demonstrate that TMZ is beneficial only in MGMT methylated tumors. However, the German NOA-08 and Nordic trials provide further evidence that TMZ is particularly beneficial in the MGMT methylated tumor subset [41]. A practical issue is whether an unspecified endpoint that is response of tumors based upon MGMT methylation status as determined in the German NOA-08 and Nordic trials changes clinical practice or even clinical trial design. It is worth mentioning that the determination of MGMT in the seminal EORTC/NCIC trail was a retrospective analysis, the results of which profoundly influenced treatment of GBM. This is particularly relevant as the NCIC/EORTC is currently conducting a randomized trial in elderly patients with GBM defined as patients >65 years of age comparing hypoRT (40 Gy in 15 fractions) with (concurrent and adjuvant) or without sdTMZ [42]. The NCIC/EORTC elderly GBM trial included MGMT promoter methylation as a prospective stratification factor. If upon completion of the trial hypoRT only is inferior therapy in elderly patients with methylated MGMT tumors, this treatment arm would then be reserved for elderly patients with unmethylated MGMT tumors assuming there is no added benefit to combination therapy in this cohort. Response based upon MGMT methylation status was never powered sufficiently in the seminal EORTC/NCIC trial to answer the question unequivocally regarding the benefit of RT + TMZ. Nonetheless, there appears to be compelling evidence that TMZ adds benefit only to the MGMT methylated cohort of newly diagnosed GBM suggesting that treatment practice changes to include MGMT methylation determination when considering either hypoRT or sdTMZ only for elderly patients

Table 5 Treatment categories of elderly patients with glioblastoma

Category	Preferred treatment
Physiologically young (geriatric scale assessment)	Hypofractionated radiotherapy in unmethylated MGMT tumors
	Standard dose temozolomide in methylated MGMT tumors
Frail with good performance	Hypofractionated radiotherapy or standard dose temozolomide only
Compromised performance	No treatment or hypofractionated radiotherapy

outside of a clinical trial. Determining a standard of care for elderly patients with newly diagnosed GBM would constitute a significant achievement and based upon the NOA-08 and Nordic trials that realization appears closer.

3 Summary

In conclusion, elderly patients with GBM appear at this juncture based upon available prospective evidence to benefit from either hypoRT or TMZ only with deferred RT (Table 5) [43]. The benefit if any of combination therapy (RT + TMZ) in the elderly will be adjudicated in the soon-to-be-completed NCIC/EORTC trial. Because determination of the tumor promoter MGMT methylation status appears both prognostic as well as predictive in the elderly, assessment of MGMT methylation is important in determining best therapy (hypoRT vs. sdTMZ) and consequently should become a standard practice in the elderly with GBM.

References

1. Stupp R, Mason WP, Van Den Bent MJ et al (2005) Radiotherapy plus concomitant and adjuvant temozolomide for glioblastoma. N Eng J Med 352(10):987–996. doi:10.1056/NEJMoa043330
2. Hess KR, Broglio KR, Bondy ML (2004) Adult glioma incidence trends in the United States, 1977–2000. Cancer 101(10):2293–2299. doi:10.1002/cncr.20621
3. Paszat L, Laperriere N, GroomeP Schulze K, Mackillop W, Holowaty E (2001) A population-based study of glioblastoma multiforme. Int J Rad Onc Biol Phys 51(1):100–107
4. Dolecek TA, Propp JM, Stroup NE, Kruchko C (2012) CBTRUS statistical report: primary brain and central nervous system tumors diagnosed in the United States in 2005–2009. Neuro Oncol 14(Suppl 5):v1–49. doi:10.1093/neuonc/nos218
5. Stupp R, Hegi Me, Mason WP et al (2009) Effects of radiotherapy with concomitant and adjuvant temozolomide versus radiotherapy alone on survival in glioblastoma in a randomized phase III study: 5-year analysis of the EORTC-NCIC trial. Lancet Oncol 10(5):459–466. doi:10.1016/S1470-2045(09)70025-70027
6. Keime-Guibert F, Chinot O, Taillandier L et al (2007) Radiotherapy for glioblastoma in the elderly. N Engl J Med 356(15):1527–1535. doi:10.1056/NEJMoa065901

7. Roa W, Brasher PM, Bauman G et al (2004) Abbreviated course of radiation therapy in older patients with glioblastoma multiforme: a prospective randomized clinical trial. J Clin Oncol 22 (9):1583–1588. doi:10.1200/JCO.2004.06.082
8. Grossman SA, Ye X, Piantadosi S et al (2010) Survival of patients with newly diagnosed glioblastoma treated with radiation and temozolomide in research studies in the United States. Clin Cancer Res 16(8):2443–2449. doi:10.1158/1078-0432.CCR-09-3106
9. Brem SS, Bierman PJ, Brem H et al (2011) Central nervous system cancers. J Natl Compr Canc Netw 9(4):352–400
10. Iwamoto FM, Reiner AS, Panageas KS, Elkin EB, Abrey LE (2008) Patterns of care in elderly glioblastoma patients. Ann Neurol 64(6):628–634. doi:10.1002/ana.21521
11. Barnholtz-Sloan JS, Williams VL, Maldonado JL, Shahani D, Stockwell HG, Chamberlain M, Sloan AE (2008) Patterns of care and outcomes among elderly individuals with primary malignant astrocytoma. J Neurosurg 108:642–648. doi:10.3171/JNS/2008/108/4/0642
12. Curran WJ Jr, Scott CB, Horton J, Nelson JS, Weinstein AS, Fischbach AJ, Chang CH, Rotman M, Asbell SO, Krisch RE (1993) Recursive partitioning analysis of prognostic factors in three Radiation Therapy Oncology Group malignant glioma trials. J Natl Cancer Inst 85 (9):704–710
13. Hegi ME, Diserens AC, Gorlia T et al (2005) MGMT gene silencing and benefit from temozolomide in glioblastoma. N Engl J Med 352(10):997–1003. doi:10.1056/NEJMoa043331
14. Toedt G, Barbus S, Wolter M et al (2011) Molecular signatures classify astrocytic gliomas by IDH1 mutation status. Int J Cancer 128(5):1095–1103. doi:10.1002/ijc.25448
15. Parsons DW, Jones S, Zhang X, Lin JC, Leary RJ, Angenendt P, Mankoo P, Carter H, Siu IM, Gallia GL et al (2008) An integrated genomic analysis of human glioblastoma multiforme. Science 321(5897):1807–1812. doi:10.1126/science.1164382
16. Yan H, Parsons DW, Jin G, McLendon R, Rasheed BA, Yuan W, Kos I, Batinic-Haberle I, Jones S, Riggins GJ et al (2009) IDH1 and IDH2 mutations in gliomas. N Engl J Med 360 (8):765–773. doi:10.1056/NEJMoa0808710
17. Hartmann C, Hentschel B, Wick W, Capper D, Felsberg J, Simon M, Westphal M, Schackert G, Meyermann R, Pietsch T et al (2010) Patients with IDH1 wild type anaplastic astrocytomas exhibit worse prognosis than IDH1-mutated glioblastomas, and IDH1 mutation status accounts for the unfavorable prognostic effect of higher age: implications for classification of gliomas. Acta Neuropathol 120(6):707–718. doi:10.1007/s00401-010-0781-z
18. Wick W, Platten M, Meisner C et al (2012) Temozolomide chemotherapy alone versus radiotherapy alone for malignant astrocytoma in the elderly: the NOA-08 randomised, phase 3 trial. Lancet Oncol 13(7):707–715. doi:10.1016/S1470-2045(12)70164-X
19. Gilbert M, Wang M, Aldape KD et al (2013) A randomized phase III trial comparing standard adjuvant temozolomide with a dose-dense schedule in newly diagnosed glioblastoma. J Clin Oncol 31(32):4085–4091. doi:10.1200/JCO.2013.49.6968
20. Reifenberger G, Hentschel B, Felsberg J, Schackert G, Simon M, Schnell O, Westphal M, Wick W, Pietsch T, Loeffler M et al (2012) Predictive impact of MGMT promoter methylation in glioblastoma of the elderly. Int J Cancer 131(6):1342–1350. doi:10.1002/ijc.27385
21. Holdhoff M, Ye X, Blakeley JO, Blair L, Burger PC, Grossman SA, Diaz LA Jr (2012) Use of personalized molecular biomarkers in the clinical care of adults with glioblastomas. J Neurooncol 110(2):279–285. doi:10.1007/s11060-012-0968-3
22. Iwamoto FM, Cooper AR, Reiner AS, Nayak L, Abrey LE (2009) Glioblastoma in the elderly: the Memorial Sloan-Kettering Cancer Center Experience (1997–2007). Cancer 115(6):3758–3766. doi:10.1002/cncr.24413
23. Balducci L, Extermann M (2000) Management of cancer in the older person: a practical approach. Oncologist 5(3):224–237. doi:10.1634/theoncologist.5-3-224
24. Kita D, Ciernik IF, Vaccarella S, Franceschi S, Kleihues P, Lutolf UM, Ohgaki H (2009) Age as a predictive factor in glioblastomas: population-based study. Neuroepidemiology 33(1):17–22. doi:10.1159/000210017
25. Paszat L, Laperriere N, Groome P, Schulze K, Mackillop W, Holowaty E (2001) A population-based study of glioblastoma multiforme. Int J Radiat Oncol Biol Phys 51(1):100–107

26. Glantz M, Chamberlain MC, Liu Q, Litofsky NS, Recht LD (2003) Temozolomide as an alternative to irradiation for elderly patients with newly diagnosed malignant gliomas. Cancer 97(9):2262–2266. doi:10.1002/cncr.11323i
27. Chamberlain MC, Chalmers L (2007) A pilot study of primary temozolomide chemotherapy and deferred radiotherapy in elderly patients with glioblastoma. J Neurooncol 82(2):207–209
28. Brada M, Stenning S, Gabe R et al (2010) Temozolomide versus procarbazine, lomustine, and vincristine in recurrent high-grade glioma. J Clinical Oncol 28(30):4601–4608. doi:10.1200/JCO.2009.27.1932
29. Malmstrom A, Gronberg BH, Marosi C, Stupp R, Frappaz D, Schultz H, Abacioglu U, Tavelin B, Lhermitte B, Hegi ME et al (2012) Temozolomide versus standard 6-week radiotherapy versus hypofractionated radiotherapy in patients older than 60 years with glioblastoma: the Nordic randomised, phase 3 trial. Lancet Oncol 13(9):916–926. doi:10.1016/S1470-2045(12)70265-6
30. Gallego P-L, Ducray F, Chinot O et al (2011) Temozolomide in elderly patients with newly diagnosed glioblastoma and poor performance status: an ANOCEF phase II trial. J Clin Oncol 29(22):3050–3055. doi:10.1200/JCO.2011.34.8086
31. Reyes-Botero G, Honnorat J, Chinot O et al. Temozolomide plus bevacizumab in elderly patients with newly diagnosed and poor performance status: An ANOCEF Phase 2 trial. J Clin Oncol 31, 2013 (suppl; abstr 2020)
32. Gilbert MR, Dignam JJ, Armstrong TS, Wefel JS et al (2014) A randomized trial of bevacizumab for newly diagnosed glioblastoma. N Engl J Med 370(8):699–708. doi:10.1056/NEJMoa1308573
33. Chinot O, Wick W, Mason W et al (2014) Bevacizumab plus radiotherapy-temozolomide for newly diagnosed glioblastoma. N Engl J Med 370(8):709–722. doi:10.1056/NEJMoa1308345
34. Sijben AE, McIntyre JB, Roldan GB, Easaw JC, Yan E, Forsyth PA, Parney IF, Magliocco AM, Bernsen H, Cairncross JG (2008) Toxicity from chemoradiotherapy in older patients with glioblastoma multiforme. J Neurooncol 89(1):97–103. doi:10.1007/s11060-008-9593-6
35. Brandes AA, Franceschi E, Tosoni A, Benevento F, Scopece L, Mazzocchi V, Bacci A, Agati R, Calbucci F, Ermani M (2009) Temozolomide concomitant and adjuvant to radiotherapy in elderly patients with glioblastoma: correlation with MGMT promoter methylation status. Cancer 115(15):3512–3518. doi:10.1002/cncr.24406
36. Minniti G, Salvati M, Arcella A, Buttarelli F, D'Elia A, Lanzetta G, Esposito V, Scarpino S, Maurizi Enrici R, Giangaspero F (2011) Correlation between O6-methylguanine-DNA methyltransferase and survival in elderly patients with glioblastoma treated with radiotherapy plus concomitant and adjuvant temozolomide. J Neurooncol 102(2):311–316. doi:10.1007/s11060-010-0324-4
37. Minniti G, De Sanctis V, Muni R, Filippone F, Bozzao A, Valeriani M, Osti MF, De Paula U, Lanzetta G, Tombolini V et al (2008) Radiotherapy plus concomitant and adjuvant temozolomide for glioblastoma in elderly patients. J Neurooncol 88(1):97–103. doi:10.1007/s11060-008-9538-0
38. Barker CA, Chang M, Chou JF, Zhang Z, Beal K, Gutin PH, Iwamoto FM (2012) Radiotherapy and concomitant temozolomide may improve survival of elderly patients with glioblastoma. J Neurooncol 109(2):391–397. doi:10.1007/s11060-012-0906-4
39. Combs SE, Wagner J, Bischof M, Welzel T, Edler L, Rausch R, Wagner F, Zabel-du Bois A, Debus J, Schulz-Ertner D (2008) Radiochemotherapy in patients with primary glioblastoma comparing two temozolomide dose regimens. Int J Radiat Oncol Biol Phys 71(4):999–1005. doi:10.1016/j.ijrobp.2007.11.064
40. Fiorica F, Berretta M, Colosimo C, Stefanelli A, Ursino S, Zanet E, Palmucci T, Maugeri D, Malaguarnera M, Palmucci S et al (2010) Glioblastoma in elderly patients: safety and efficacy of adjuvant radiotherapy with concomitant temozolomide. Arch Gerontol Geriatr 51(1):31–35. doi:10.1016/j.archger.2009.06.011
41. Tanaka S, Meyer FB, Buckner JC, Uhm JH, Yan ES, Parney IF (2013) Presentation, management, and outcome of newly diagnosed glioblastoma in elderly patients. J Neurosurg 118(4):786–798. doi:10.3171/2012.10.JNS112268

42. Laperriere N, Weller M, Stupp R, Perry JR, Brandes AA, Wick W, van den Bent MJ (2013) Optimal management of elderly patients with glioblastoma. Cancer Treat Rev 39(4):350–357. doi:10.1016/j.ctrv.2012.05.008
43. Perry JR, Callaghan CO, Ding K et al (2012) A phase III randomized controlled trial of short-course radiotherapy with or without concomitant and adjuvant temozolomide in elderly patients with glioblastoma (NCIC CTG CE.6, EORTC 26062-22061, TROG 08.02). Can J Neuro Sci 39(1):16

Palliative and Supportive Care for Glioma Patients

Tobias Walbert and Kristen Chasteen

Abstract The diagnosis of a brain tumor is a life-changing event for patients and families. High-grade gliomas are incurable and long-term survival remains limited. While low-grade glioma patients have better outcomes, their quality of life is often affected by a variety of symptoms as well. Helping glioma patients improve quality of life at all stages of illness is an important goal for the interdisciplinary care team. There is evidence from advanced lung cancer patients that early involvement of a palliative care team can improve patient's quality of life, symptom burden, and even survival and a similar approach benefits glioma patients as well. Patients with high-grade and low-grade glioma often suffer from significant symptom burden. We discuss how validated global symptom assessments and symptom-specific screening tools are useful to identify distressing symptoms. Seizures, fatigue, depression, and anxiety are some of the more common symptoms throughout the disease course and should be managed actively. Patients with glioma also have high symptom burden at the end of life and the majority lose decision-making capacity. Advance care planning conversations early in the disease course are essential to elicit the patient's wishes for end of life care and effective communication with surrogate decision makers during all stages of the disease helps ensure that those wishes are respected.

Keywords Glioma · Symptom management · End-of-life · Supportive care · Palliative care · Glioblastoma · Glioma

Contents

T. Walbert (✉) · K. Chasteen
Departments of Neurosurgery and Neurology, Henry Ford Health System,
2799 W Grand Blvd, Detroit, MI 48202, USA
e-mail: twalber1@hfhs.org

J. Raizer and A. Parsa (eds.), *Current Understanding and Treatment of Gliomas*,
Cancer Treatment and Research 163, DOI 10.1007/978-3-319-12048-5_11

1 Introduction

The diagnosis of a brain tumor is a life-changing event for patients and their families.

Glioblastomas (GBMs) and the majority of anaplastic gliomas are treated with maximal surgical resection, followed by radiotherapy with concurrent and adjuvant chemotherapy to the residual tumor and the surrounding brain tissue. Despite this aggressive approach, long-term survival remains limited for most patients with high-grade glioma and even those with low-grade glioma often suffer from significant neurologic complications of their disease [1–3].

While the primary treatment is geared to extend life and progression-free survival, there is increasing appreciation by patients, families, and practitioners that maintaining quality of life is as important as increasing survival time.

Brain tumors can present with many signs and symptoms that have immediate impact on the patients' daily lives. These symptoms can be either caused by the location of the brain tumor or by oncologic treatment (surgery, radiation treatment, chemotherapy). Active symptom management is essential to not only maintain the patient's quality of life but to support caregivers and families as well. Patients' symptoms and needs might change during the course of the disease. Therefore proactive and continuous assessment of physical and psychological symptoms is important to identify those needs. Besides clinical observations, this can be done with the help of multidimensional patient-reported outcome tools [4]. Outcome measures developed specifically for brain tumor patients include quality of life measures such as the EORTC QLQ30 general measure in combination with the BN20–brain tumor module or the more symptom-assessment-focused M.D. Anderson Symptom Inventory-Brain Tumor (MDASIBT). The MDASI-BT was developed specifically to measure multiple symptoms and to assess the symptom burden in the brain tumor [5].

Neurooncologists with a background in neurology are well prepared to manage many of the neurological symptoms inflicted by brain tumors such as seizures, pain, focal weakness, and cognitive impairment; however, it is clearly understood that brain tumor patients require a multidisciplinary team approach that in addition to neurooncologists involves neurosurgeons, radiation and medical oncologists, and physiatrists and specialists in behavioral health and palliative care (PC). Given the limited survival and complex symptom burden of high-grade glioma patients, it has been proposed that the involvement of PC and hospice specialists might benefit these patients [6–8]. PC offers a proactive and systematic approach to manage symptoms

Table 1 Goals of palliative care [76]

The goals of palliative care include:
• Provides relief from pain and other distressing symptoms
• Affirms life and regards dying as a normal process
• Intends neither to hasten or postpone death
• Integrates the psychological and spiritual aspects of patient care
• Offers a support system to help patients live as actively as possible until death
• Offers a support system to help the family cope during the patients illness and in their own bereavement
• Uses a team approach to address the needs of patients and their families, including bereavement counselling, if indicated
• Will enhance quality of life, and may also positively influence the course of illness
• Is applicable early in the course of illness, in conjunction with other therapies that are intended to prolong life, such as chemotherapy or radiation therapy, and includes those investigations needed to better understand and manage distressing clinical complications

and to provide an additional layer of support to patients with serious illness (Table 1). PC should be differentiated from hospice medicine which focuses strictly on the end-of-life phase. PC is appropriate at any stage in a serious illness, can be provided along with curative treatment and is not restricted to end-of-life care.

Recently there has been new evidence that the early involvement of PC might improve symptom detection and management and have a positive impact on the psychosocial support and end-of-life planning in oncology patients [9]. A recent single-center, nonblinded randomized controlled trial investigated the role of early referral to PC in the care of patients with metastatic nonsmall cell lung cancer [10]. Patients who received early integrated outpatient PC and met frequently with a PC team had meaningful improvements in quality of life and symptom burden as well as mood. In addition, these patients received improved end-of-life care and had prolonged survival when compared to patients undergoing standard of care.

However, most brain tumor patients are referred to PC after exhausting all therapeutic options (median of 28–70 days prior to death) [7, 11, 12]. At this point, it is unclear if such an intervention would be equally beneficial for patients with brain tumors given the difference in disease and symptom profile.

2 Symptom Management in Brain Tumors

2.1 Seizures

Epileptic seizures are common in patients with brain tumors and affect between 30–80 % of all patients with brain tumors [13]. Seizures can be potentially life threatening and can cause significant morbidity especially in patients with otherwise controlled tumors [14]. The seizure frequency in patients with glioma is generally higher in low-grade (WHO grade II) tumors (60–80 %) and less prevalent in glioblastoma (WHO grade IV) (29–49 %) [13]. Generally, patients with low-grade glioma and location in the temporal lobe, parietal lobe, or cortex are at greater risk for seizures than those with tumors in the infratentorial or white matter location. About 40 % of brain tumor patients present with a seizure as a first symptom and these patients remain at an increased risk for recurrent seizures despite treatment with antiepileptic drugs (AEDs) [15]. Despite good seizure control during treatment, up to 86 % of patients suffer from seizures at the end of life [16].

The use of antiepileptic prophylaxis for glioma patients has been investigated in multiple, mostly retrospective studies [17–20] and is currently not recommended for patients who have never had a seizure [15]. AED should be tapered off 1 week after surgery, if a patient has never had a seizure [15].

Once a patient with a brain tumor has had a seizure, long-term treatment with an AED should be strongly considered as these patients are at increased risk for seizure recurrence. It is important to consider the pharmacokinetic interactions of AEDs with anticancer therapeutics. A number of older AEDs such as phenobarbital, phenytoin, primidone, carbamazepine, and oxcarbazepine induce the cytochrome 450 (CYP450) -dependent hepatic enzymes and consequently increase their own metabolism and influence the metabolism and efficacy of many commonly used cytotoxic agents. In addition, these CYP450 inducers might affect the effectiveness of dexamethasone, which utilizes the same metabolic mechanism [21]. Valproic acid, however, is a CYP450 inhibitor that might increase therapeutic drug levels of antineoplastic agents and might have other antineoplastic properties. There have been several reports of the in vitro as well as in vivo antineoplastic activity of this histone deacetylase inhibiting antiseizure medication (reviewed in Weller et al.) [22]. A retrospective (and unfortunately insufficiently powered) analysis of patients participating in the EORTC/NCIC temozolomide trial for glioblastoma revealed prolonged survival with use of valproic acid [23]. On the other hand, another retrospective analysis of patients in the North Central Cancer Treatment Group trial came to the opposite conclusion. In that study, patients taking enzyme-inducing AEDs had increased survival [24]. Currently, the true impact of valproic acid on brain tumor survival remains unclear.

Newer AEDs such as levetiracetam, lacosamide, and zonisamide are not influenced by CYP450 and other metabolic pathways and therefore do not interact with other agents utilizing these pathways. Side effects are more frequent and pronounced in brain tumor patients when compared to the general epilepsy population [15, 25]. In the setting of brain tumor patients undergoing active treatment, levetiracetam is the most studied of the newer generation antiepileptic medications. According to several studies it has been well tolerated and safe, but possible side effects include neurocognitive deficits and psychiatric effects [26, 27].

Seizure management in the end-of-life phase of brain tumor patients is crucial given the high frequency and the fact that epileptic events have been associated with nonpeaceful death [28]. The optimization in this setting is challenging due to the fact that many brain tumor patients are unable to swallow or to take oral medications due to changes in mental status [8]. If oral or intravenous application is not warranted, a number of seizure medications can be supplied intramuscularly, subcutaneously, rectally, or via buccal or intranasal application (See Anderson et al. for details) [29].

Diazepam especially can be delivered as rectal suppository and the buccal or intranasal application of midazolam has also been shown to stop seizures [30]. All these recommendations are either extrapolated from other studies or follow general guidelines for the treatment of seizures as there are no prospective trials investigating seizure management in the end-of-life phase of glioma patients.

2.2 *Fatigue*

Fatigue is defined as a persistent sensation of physical, cognitive, or emotional tiredness that is not linked to any recent activity and that impairs normal function [31]. Fatigue is a well-recognized problem in oncology and is a prevalent as well as impairing symptom in brain tumor patients [32]. Patients report impairment due to fatigue throughout the course of the disease, but it is most prevalent at the time of radiation therapy. More than 80 % of patients with primary brain tumors report fatigue at the time of radiation therapy [33]. Symptoms especially appear to increase toward the end of the 6-week radiation treatment and can last after radiation has been discontinued. Fatigue is not strictly related to tumor grade and one study showed that 39 % of patients with a low-grade glioma continued to report severe fatigue more than 8 years after finishing therapy [34]. While the exact mechanism for cancer-associated fatigue remains unclear, factors associated with a higher risk for fatigue include older age, female sex, decreased performance status, and treatment-related factors [32, 35–37].

All patients with fatigue should undergo screening for depression, which can affect between 16–39 % of patients with brain tumors [38]. Prior to initiating any fatigue-specific treatment, factors such as pain, anemia, sleep issues, metabolic problems such as thyroid dysfunction and low Vitamin D and Vitamin B12 levels, and malnutrition should be ruled out. A critical review of the patient's medication list should be performed as some frequently used medications such as antiseizure medications and corticosteroid taper are also known to cause symptoms similar to cancer-induced fatigue. After addressing these factors, general strategies to manage fatigue should be implemented (please see Armstrong TS et al. for an excellent review) [35]. Patients are encouraged to implement energy conservation techniques such as prioritization of activities and delegation of more energy intensive activities. Extensive naps during the day should be avoided to maintain the normal sleep cycle. A variety of nonpharmacological interventions have been evaluated in other solid tumors such as breast cancer. Unfortunately, there is a lack of validated interventions for brain tumor-associated fatigue and especially exercise-based regimens are often of limited value due to focal neurological deficits. Two large meta-analyses of randomized controlled trials evaluating exercise for cancer-related fatigue came to the conclusion that exercise resulted in clinically relevant improvement and might be effective in treating fatigue [39, 40]. Successful exercise programs included a focus on walking or resistance training which can only be applied to a select group of brain tumor patients without paralysis or weakness. Other nonpharmacologic interventions might include psychosocial programs focusing on education, stress management, or cognitive-behavioral interventions [40].

Integrative medicine approaches such as yoga have been successfully employed in lowering self-reported levels of fatigue [41] and in another study had a positive impact on inflammation markers, fatigue and vitality [42]. The use of acupuncture is also frequently mentioned by patients, but conclusive data describing the impact on cancer-related fatigue remains lacking [43, 44].

Many pharmacologic interventions such as hemopoietic growth factors, corticosteroids, antidepressants, and psychostimulants have been evaluated in the general solid tumor population, but only the use of stimulants such as methylphenidate and modafinil have been evaluated specifically in glioma patients [35, 45]. While earlier open-label studies with methylphenidate and modafanil showed promising cognitive and functional improvement [46, 47], later randomized-blinded trials were not able to duplicate these findings [48, 49].

Fatigue is a prevalent and disabling symptom in primary brain tumor patients with high impact on function and quality of life. Due to the lack of conclusive data for brain tumor patients, interventions must be chosen individually with consideration of possible side effects.

3 Depression and Anxiety

Depression and anxiety are recognized as frequent and distressing symptoms for patients with glioma. Estimated prevalence of depression in glioma patients is 15–39 % and anxiety 30–48 % [6, 38, 50]. Functional impairment, prior history of depression, and female sex are identified as possible risk factors for depression in patients with glioma [6, 38, 50]. Anxiety is also associated with prior history of psychiatric illness and female sex [6]. Depression and anxiety are negatively associated with quality of life, and there is a weak association between depression and reduced survival [6, 38]. The etiologies of depression and anxiety in glioma are unknown. There is no convincing evidence to support the hypothesis that tumor or surgery are direct causes of depression [51].

Diagnosing depression in patients with glioma is challenging since many of the symptoms in DSM-IV diagnostic criteria for major depressive disorder [52] (appetite change, sleep change, fatigue, poor concentration, and psychomotor slowing) could be caused by depression or by glioma and its treatment [51]. In patients who describe depressed mood or anhedonia, the safest approach is to assume that other more ambiguous symptoms are also due to depression until proven otherwise [51, 53]. Depression can also be difficult to distinguish from normal grief associated with a terminal illness. Hopelessness, worthlessness, guilt, anhedonia, and active suicidal ideation are useful in distinguishing depression from normal grief [53]. The sadness associated with normal grief also tends to come in waves rather than the pervasive sadness of depression [51]. As an adjunct to the global symptom assessment tools, the Patient Health Questionnaire-9 (PHQ-9) and the Hospital Anxiety and Depression Scale-Depression Subscale (HAD-D) have both been partially validated for use as screening tools for depression in patients with glioma [54]. Given low positive predictive value of screening, a clinical interview with collateral information from caregivers is the best way to make the diagnosis of depression [51].

There is less guidance for screening and diagnosis of anxiety in glioma patients. A single question, "How anxious have you felt this week?" and the Hospital Anxiety and Depression Scale (HAD) have both been validated as useful screening tools in cancer patients, followed by clinical interview to make a specific diagnosis [55].

There are no published randomized controlled trials of pharmacologic treatment to provide guidance in treatment of depression or anxiety in glioma [56]. Based on evidence in other seriously ill patients and cancer patients [55, 57, 58], selective serotonin reuptake inhibitors (SSRIs) may be considered as first-line therapy for treatment of depression [51] and anxiety in glioma patients. Slow titration to therapeutic doses and monitoring for drug–drug interactions is advised [55]. There are no prospective data about the safety of SSRIs in glioma patients; however, retrospective studies have not shown increased toxicity [51]. Unlike bupropion, clomipramine, high or moderate dose tricyclics, and venlafaxine, SSRIs are also a good choice for glioma patients as they are not associated with increased seizure risk in the general population [59, 60]. There is evidence to support the use of benzodiazepines as effective short-term treatment of anxiety in cancer patients [55], but they should be used cautiously given the increased risk of delirium [61]. Psychotherapy may have beneficial impacts on symptoms of depression and anxiety in patients with other systemic cancers [55]; however, the benefit and feasibility in glioma patients is unknown [51].

4 End-of-Life Care in Brain Tumor Patients

High-grade glioma remains incurable and long-term survival is very limited. Two recent systematic reviews have investigated symptoms of brain tumor patients in the end-of-life phase [8, 62] and show that patients suffer from a consistently high symptom burden [7, 11, 28, 63–65]. Cognitive disturbances, delirium, somnolence, and aphasia are common with progressive high-grade glioma [62]. The majority of patients with high-grade glioma lack decision-making capacity in the last month of life and this capacity decreases even more during the last week before death [12, 28, 66]. Therefore, advance care planning conversations early in the disease course are essential [8, 62]. Relatives of glioma patients identified absence of transitions between settings as an important factor in allowing the patient to have a dignified death [67]. Advance care planning helps ensure that end-of-life care matches preferred care [68] and may help avoid burdensome transitions at the end of life. Completion of an

Table 2 Early advance care planning conversations—“PAUSE” [77]

P	Pause in the work of the visit	Take a moment to prepare to introduce this part of the conversation.
		“There is something I’d like to put on our agenda today”
A	Ask permission to raise the issue	“Could we take a moment to talk about what we should do if you get a lot sicker?”
U	Understand big-picture values	“Have you heard about advance directives or living wills?”
		“If this disease was getting worse and it looked like time was short, what would be most important to you?”
S	Suggest a surrogate	“Have you thought about who would be the best person to make medical decisions if you were too sick to make them yourself?”
E	Expect emotion and emphasize	“This can be tough to talk about”
		“It can be scary to think about things not going well”

advance directive is an important part of advance care planning, but it is not sufficient to ensure that patients’ wishes are respected. One study found that in 40 % of glioma patients, physicians were unaware of the patients’ end-of-life preferences, even though several had an advanced directive according to their relatives [66]. This data highlights the importance of not just completing a document, but also discussing plans with the family and the healthcare team. It also serves as a reminder to clinicians to ask about patients’ care preferences and advance directives.

There are few studies focusing specifically on interventions to improve advance care planning for patients with high-grade glioma [62]. In one study, patients with high-grade glioma who watched a video decision support tool were more likely to avoid CPR [69]. The most effective way to integrate early advance care planning into the care of all patients with high-grade glioma is unknown and it can be difficult to find time for advance care planning during busy clinic visits. A helpful roadmap for advance care planning conversations early in the course of serious illness is outlined by the acronym “PAUSE” (Table 2) [77]. The goal of the “PAUSE” roadmap is to allow clinicians to assess whether or not the patient is ready to discuss advance care planning, begin to understand their goals, encourage assigning a surrogate decision maker, and provide emotional support. The conversation may need to be continued with another member of the interdisciplinary team or at the next clinic visit.

4.1 Later Goals of Care Discussions

Another communication challenge that clinicians who care for patients with glioma face is navigating discussions about goals of care when the disease has progressed and the burdens of further anticancer therapy are beginning to outweigh the benefits. When oncologists discuss the possibility of discontinuing chemotherapy, they often have feelings of guilt and failure that they were unable to rescue the patient from

Table 3 Addressing goals of care for patients late in the disease course (often done with a surrogate decision maker)—"REMAP" [77]

R	Reframe why the status quo isn't working	You may need to discuss serious news (e.g., a scan result) first
		"Given this news, it seems like a good time to talk about what to do now"
E	Expect emotion and empathize	"I can see you're worried"
		"Tell me more about that—what are you concerned about?"
		"Is it ok for us to talk about what this means?"
M	Map goals and values	"If your wife could participate in this discussion, what would she say?"
		"Did your wife ever talk about what we should do if she got a lot sicker?"
		For patients: "Thinking of the time ahead, what is most important to you?"
A	Align with patient's values	As i listen to you, it sounds like the most important things are [x, y, z]
P	Plan treatments that match patient values	Here's what I can do now that will help your wife get the kind of care she said she wanted. What do you think about it?
EXTRA	Expect questions about more treatments	Here are the pros and cons of what you are asking about
		Overall, my experience tells me that more [x] would do more harm than good at this point
EXTRA	Talk about services that would help before introducing the word hospice	We've talked about wanting to get more help for you at home to manage your wife's seizures so she doesn't have to come to the emergency room
		One thing that can help is having a team come to your house to provide extra support. The team that could offer the most support is hospice

impending death [70]. In addition many clinicians worry that discussing end-of-life care will take away hope; however, most patients want detailed information about their illness and what to expect [71]. Patients and families do want clinicians to convey empathy, support, and hope [72]. It is helpful to realize that an entire spectrum of hope can exist and evolve over time, including hope for cure, hope for living longer, hope for having time with loved ones, and hope for having a peaceful death [73]. Patients want to establish relationships with clinicians who see them as individuals [74], and want to trust clinicians with whom they discuss end-of-life concerns [75]. A useful roadmap to meet these patient and family needs in discussing goals of care late in the disease course is outlined by the acronym "REMAP" [77]. (Table 3) For patients with glioma, these later conversations will likely often occur with surrogate decision makers. A key skill is to ask questions to elicit the patient's big-picture values prior to discussing specific treatment plans like stopping chemotherapy or enrolling in hospice care [70], e.g., "Did your wife ever talk about what we should do if she got a lot sicker and it looked like time was short?" Eliciting the patient's values will then allow clinicians to recommend a care plan that is tailored to meet the patient's goals.

5 Conclusion

Many patients with glioma have very limited life expectancies and may suffer from high symptom burden. Interventions to improve quality of life should be a focus of care along with life-extending therapies at all stages of illness. Seizures, fatigue, depression, and anxiety are some of the common distressing symptoms that can occur. There are validated global assessment tools and more specific symptom assessment tools that can be used for initial screening in all patients with glioma. Unfortunately, there is a lack of studies evaluating specific strategies to control symptoms and improve life in this patient population. Extrapolating the data from studies performed in other cancer patients may help direct management. In addition to symptom management, effective communication is also essential to promoting quality of life in patients with glioma. Since the majority of glioma patients lack decision-making capabilities in the last month of life, advance care planning conversations early in the disease course are essential. Effective communication with surrogate decision makers during the later stages of the disease helps ensure that the patient's wishes are respected.

Funding Department of Neurosurgery and the Hermelin Brain Tumor Center, Henry Ford Health System.

Conflict of Interest There are no conflicts of interest to declare.

References

1. Prados MD, Seiferheld W, Sandler HM et al (2004) Phase III randomized study of radiotherapy plus procarbazine, lomustine, and vincristine with or without BUdR for treatment of anaplastic astrocytoma: final report of RTOG 9404. Int J Radiat Oncol Biol Phys 58:1147–1152
2. Stupp R, Mason WP, van den Bent MJ et al (2005) Radiotherapy plus concomitant and adjuvant temozolomide for glioblastoma. N Engl J Med 352:987–996
3. van den Bent MJ, Carpentier AF, Brandes AA et al (2006) Adjuvant procarbazine, lomustine, and vincristine improves progression-free survival but not overall survival in newly diagnosed anaplastic oligodendrogliomas and oligoastrocytomas: a randomized European Organisation for Research and Treatment of Cancer phase III trial. J Clin Oncol 24:2715–2722

4. Armstrong TS (2013) Measuring clinical benefit: use of patient-reported outcomes (PRO) in primary brain tumor clinical trials. Curr Oncol Rep 15:27–32
5. Armstrong TS, Mendoza T, Gning I et al (2006) Validation of the MD Anderson symptom inventory brain tumor module (MDASI-BT). J Neurooncol 80:27–35
6. Ford E, Catt S, Chalmers A, Fallowfield L (2012) Systematic review of supportive care needs in patients with primary malignant brain tumors. Neurooncology 14:392–404
7. Gofton TE, Graber J, Carver A (2012) Identifying the palliative care needs of patients living with cerebral tumors and metastases: a retrospective analysis. J Neurooncol 108:527–534
8. Walbert T, Khan M (2014) End-of-life symptoms and care in patients with primary malignant brain tumors: a systematic literature review. J Neurooncol 117(2):217–224
9. Greer JA, Jackson VA, Meier DE, Temel JS (2013) Early integration of palliative care services with standard oncology care for patients with advanced cancer. CA Cancer J Clin 63:349–363
10. Temel JS, Greer JA, Muzikansky A et al (2010) Early palliative care for patients with metastatic non-small-cell lung cancer. N Engl J Med 363:733–742
11. Arber A, Faithfull S, Plaskota M, Lucas C, de Vries K (2010) A study of patients with a primary malignant brain tumour and their carers: symptoms and access to services. Int J Palliat Nurs 16:24–30
12. Oberndorfer S, Lindeck-Pozza E, Lahrmann H, Struhal W, Hitzenberger P, Grisold W (2008) The end-of-life hospital setting in patients with glioblastoma. J Palliat Med 11:26–30
13. van Breemen MS, Wilms EB, Vecht CJ (2007) Epilepsy in patients with brain tumours: epidemiology, mechanisms, and management. Lancet Neurol 6:421–430
14. Taphoorn MJ (2003) Neurocognitive sequelae in the treatment of low-grade gliomas. Semin Oncol 30:45–48
15. Glantz MJ, Cole BF, Forsyth PA et al (2000) Practice parameter: anticonvulsant prophylaxis in patients with newly diagnosed brain tumors. Report of the Quality Standards Subcommittee of the American Academy of Neurology. Neurology 54:1886–1893
16. Pace A, Villani V, Di Lorenzo C et al (2013) Epilepsy in the end-of-life phase in patients with high-grade gliomas. J Neurooncol 111:83–86
17. Ansari SF, Bohnstedt BN, Perkins SM, Althouse SK, Miller JC (2014) Efficacy of postoperative seizure prophylaxis in intra-axial brain tumor resections. J Neurooncol 118 (1):117–122
18. Mahaley MS Jr, Dudka L (1981) The role of anticonvulsant medications in the management of patients with anaplastic gliomas. Surg Neurol 16:399–401
19. North JB, Penhall RK, Hanieh A, Frewin DB, Taylor WB (1983) Phenytoin and postoperative epilepsy: a double-blind study. J Neurosurg 58:672–677
20. Wu AS, Trinh VT, Suki D et al (2013) A prospective randomized trial of perioperative seizure prophylaxis in patients with intraparenchymal brain tumors. J Neurosurg 118:873–883
21. Vecht CJ, Wagner GL, Wilms EB (2003) Interactions between antiepileptic and chemotherapeutic drugs. Lancet Neurol 2:404–409
22. Weller M, Stupp R, Wick W (2012) Epilepsy meets cancer: when, why, and what to do about it? Lancet Oncol 13:e375–e382
23. Weller M, Gorlia T, Cairncross JG et al (2011) Prolonged survival with valproic acid use in the EORTC/NCIC temozolomide trial for glioblastoma. Neurology 77:1156–1164
24. Jaeckle KA, Ballman K, Furth A, Buckner JC (2009) Correlation of enzyme-inducing anticonvulsant use with outcome of patients with glioblastoma. Neurology 73:1207–1213
25. Moots PL, Maciunas RJ, Eisert DR, Parker RA, Laporte K, Abou-Khalil B (1995) The course of seizure disorders in patients with malignant gliomas. Arch Neurol 52:717–724
26. Maschio M, Dinapoli L, Sperati F et al (2012) Oxcarbazepine monotherapy in patients with brain tumor-related epilepsy: open-label pilot study for assessing the efficacy, tolerability and impact on quality of life. J Neurooncol 106:651–656
27. Usery JB, Michael LM 2nd, Sills AK, Finch CK (2010) A prospective evaluation and literature review of levetiracetam use in patients with brain tumors and seizures. J Neurooncol 99:251–260

28. Bausewein C, Hau P, Borasio GDI, Voltz R (2003) How do patients with primary brain tumours die? Palliat Med 17:558–559
29. Anderson GD, Saneto RP (2012) Current oral and non-oral routes of antiepileptic drug delivery. Adv Drug Deliv Rev 64:911–918
30. Nakken KO, Lossius MI (2011) Buccal midazolam or rectal diazepam for treatment of residential adult patients with serial seizures or status epilepticus. Acta Neurol Scand 124:99–103
31. Berger AM, Abernethy AP, Atkinson A et al (2010) Cancer-related fatigue. J Natl Compr Canc Netw 8:904–931
32. Armstrong TS, Cron SG, Bolanos EV, Gilbert MR, Kang DH (2010) Risk factors for fatigue severity in primary brain tumor patients. Cancer 116:2707–2715
33. Lovely MP, Miaskowski C, Dodd M (1999) Relationship between fatigue and quality of life in patients with glioblastoma multiformae. Oncol Nurs Forum 26:921–925
34. Struik K, Klein M, Heimans JJ et al (2009) Fatigue in low-grade glioma. J Neurooncol 92:73–78
35. Armstrong TS, Gilbert MR (2012) Practical strategies for management of fatigue and sleep disorders in people with brain tumors. Neurooncology 14(Suppl 4):iv65–iv72
36. Faithfull S, Brada M (1998) Somnolence syndrome in adults following cranial irradiation for primary brain tumours. Clin Oncol (R Coll Radiol) 10:250–254
37. Habets EJ, Taphoorn MJ, Nederend S et al (2014) Health-related quality of life and cognitive functioning in long-term anaplastic oligodendroglioma and oligoastrocytoma survivors. J Neurooncol 116:161–168
38. Rooney AG, Carson A, Grant R (2011) Depression in cerebral glioma patients: a systematic review of observational studies. J Natl Cancer Inst 103:61–76
39. Cramp F, Daniel J (2008) Exercise for the management of cancer-related fatigue in adults. Cochrane Database Syst Rev 2(2):CD006145
40. Kangas M, Bovbjerg DH, Montgomery GH (2008) Cancer-related fatigue: a systematic and meta-analytic review of non-pharmacological therapies for cancer patients. Psychol Bull 134:700–741
41. Chandwani KD, Perkins G, Nagendra HR et al (2014) Randomized, controlled trial of yoga in women with breast cancer undergoing tadiotherapy. J Clin Oncol 32(10):1058–1065
42. Kiecolt-Glaser JK, Bennett JM, Andridge R et al (2014) Yoga's impact on inflammation, mood, and fatigue in breast cancer survivors: a randomized controlled trial. J Clin Oncol
43. Posadzki P, Moon TW, Choi TY, Park TY, Lee MS, Ernst E (2013) Acupuncture for cancer-related fatigue: a systematic review of randomized clinical trials. Support Care Cancer 21:2067–2073
44. Zeng Y, Luo T, Finnegan-John J, Cheng AS (2013) Meta-analysis of randomized controlled trials of acupuncture for cancer-related fatigue. Integr Cancer Ther 13(3):193–200
45. Boele FW, Klein M, Reijneveld JC, Verdonck-de Leeuw IM, Heimans JJ (2014) Symptom management and quality of life in glioma patients. Future Medicine 3:37–47
46. Meyers CA, Weitzner MA, Valentine AD, Levin VA (1998) Methylphenidate therapy improves cognition, mood, and function of brain tumor patients. J Clin Oncol 16:2522–2527
47. Gehring K, Patwardhan SY, Collins R et al (2012) A randomized trial on the efficacy of methylphenidate and modafinil for improving cognitive functioning and symptoms in patients with a primary brain tumor. J Neurooncol 107:165–174
48. Boele FW, Douw L, de Groot M et al (2013) The effect of modafinil on fatigue, cognitive functioning, and mood in primary brain tumor patients: a multicenter randomized controlled trial. Neurooncology 15:1420–1428
49. Butler JM Jr, Case LD, Atkins J et al (2007) A phase III, double-blind, placebo-controlled prospective randomized clinical trial of d-threo-methylphenidate HCl in brain tumor patients receiving radiation therapy. Int J Radiat Oncol Biol Phys 69:1496–1501
50. Rooney AG, McNamara S, Mackinnon M et al (2013) The frequency, longitudinal course, clinical associations, and causes of emotional distress during primary treatment of cerebral glioma. Neurooncology 15:635–643

51. Rooney AG, Brown PD, Reijneveld JC, Grant R (2014) Depression in glioma: a primer for clinicians and researchers. J Neurol Neurosurg Psychiatry 85:230–235
52. Association AP (2000) Diagnostic and statistical manual of mental disorders, 4th edn. Washington, DC
53. Block SD (2006) Psychological issues in end-of-life care. J Palliat Med 9:751–772
54. Rooney AG, McNamara S, Mackinnon M et al (2013) Screening for major depressive disorder in adults with cerebral glioma: an initial validation of 3 self-report instruments. Neurooncology 15:122–129
55. Traeger L, Greer JA, Fernandez-Robles C, Temel JS, Pirl WF (2012) Evidence-based treatment of anxiety in patients with cancer. J Clin Oncol 30:1197–1205
56. Rooney A, Grant R (2013) Pharmacological treatment of depression in patients with a primary brain tumour. Cochrane Database Syst Rev 5:CD006932
57. Rayner L, Price A, Evans A, Valsraj K, Higginson IJ, Hotopf M (2010) Antidepressants for depression in physically ill people. Cochrane Database Syst Rev:CD007503
58. Rayner L, Price A, Evans A, Valsraj K, Hotopf M, Higginson IJ (2011) Antidepressants for the treatment of depression in palliative care: systematic review and meta-analysis. Palliat Med 25:36–51
59. Alldredge BK (1999) Seizure risk associated with psychotropic drugs: clinical and pharmacokinetic considerations. Neurology 53:S68–75
60. Alper K, Schwartz KA, Kolts RL, Khan A (2007) Seizure incidence in psychopharmacological clinical trials: an analysis of Food and Drug Administration (FDA) summary basis of approval reports. Biol Psychiatry 62:345–354
61. LeGrand SB (2012) Delirium in palliative medicine: a review. J Pain Symptom Manage 44:583–594
62. Sizoo EM, Pasman HR, Dirven L et al (2014) The end-of-life phase of high-grade glioma patients: a systematic review. Support Care Cancer 22:847–857
63. Faithfull S, Cook K, Lucas C (2005) Palliative care of patients with a primary malignant brain tumour: case review of service use and support provided. Palliat Med 19:545–550
64. Pace A, Di Lorenzo C, Lorenzo CD et al (2009) End of life issues in brain tumor patients. J Neurooncol 91:39–43
65. Sizoo EM, Braam L, Postma TJ et al (2010) Symptoms and problems in the end-of-life phase of high-grade glioma patients. Neurooncology 12:1162–1166
66. Sizoo EM, Pasman HRW, Buttolo J et al (2012) Decision-making in the end-of-life phase of high-grade glioma patients. Eur J Cancer 48:226–232
67. Sizoo EM, Taphoorn MJ, Uitdehaag B et al (2013) The end-of-Life phase of high-grade glioma patients: dying with dignity? Oncologist 18:198–203
68. Houben CH, Spruit MA, Groenen MT, Wouters EF, Janssen DJ (2014) Efficacy of advance care planning: a systematic review and meta-analysis. J Am Med Dir Assoc
69. El-Jawahri A, Podgurski LM, Eichler AF et al (2010) Use of video to facilitate end-of-life discussions with patients with cancer: a randomized controlled trial. J Clin Oncol 28:305–310
70. Back AL, Arnold RM, Baile WF, Tulsky JA, Fryer-Edwards K (2005) Approaching difficult communication tasks in oncology. CA Cancer J Clin 55:164–177
71. Parker SM, Clayton JM, Hancock K et al (2007) A systematic review of prognostic/end-of-life communication with adults in the advanced stages of a life-limiting illness: patient/caregiver preferences for the content, style, and timing of information. J Pain Symptom Manage 34:81–93
72. Clayton JM, Hancock KM, Butow PN, et al (2007) Clinical practice guidelines for communicating prognosis and end-of-life issues with adults in the advanced stages of a life-limiting illness, and their caregivers. Med J Aust 186(12 Suppl):S77–S79, S83–108
73. Back AL, Anderson WG, Bunch L et al (2008) Communication about cancer near the end of life. Cancer 113:1897–1910
74. Wright EB, Holcombe C, Salmon P (2004) Doctors' communication of trust, care, and respect in breast cancer: qualitative study. BMJ 328:864

75. Walczak A, Butow PN, Davidson PM et al (2013) Patient perspectives regarding communication about prognosis and end-of-life issues: how can it be optimised? Patient Educ Couns 90:307–314
76. World Health Organization (2014) Programmes and projects: cancer control. Policies and managerial guidelines. http://www.who.int/cancer/palliative/definition/en. Accessed 03 Oct 2014
77. Arnold R, Back A, Edwards K, et al (2014) www.vitaltalk.org. Accessed 03 Oct 2014

MIX
Papier aus verantwortungsvollen Quellen
Paper from responsible sources
FSC® C105338

If you have any concerns about our products,
you can contact us on
ProductSafety@springernature.com

In case Publisher is established outside the EU,
the EU authorized representative is:
Springer Nature Customer Service Center GmbH
Europaplatz 3, 69115 Heidelberg, Germany

Printed by Libri Plureos GmbH
in Hamburg, Germany